# Frontiers in Occupational Health and Safety

## (*Volume 2*)

### *Introduction to Occupational Health Hazards*

**Edited by**

**Farhana Zahir**

*Prism Educational Society, Aligarh, U.P., India*

# Frontiers in Occupational Health and Safety

*Volume # 2*

*Introduction to Occupational Health Hazards*

Editor: Farhana Zahir

ISSN (Online): 2352-9431

ISSN (Print): 2352-9423

ISBN (Online): 978-981-14-0691-1

ISBN (Print): 978-981-14-0690-4

© 2019, Bentham eBooks imprint.

Published by Bentham Science Publishers Pte. Ltd. Singapore. All Rights Reserved.

need for a court order if at any point you breach any terms of this License Agreement. In no event will any delay or failure by Bentham Science Publishers in enforcing your compliance with this License Agreement constitute a waiver of any of its rights.

3. You acknowledge that you have read this License Agreement, and agree to be bound by its terms and conditions. To the extent that any other terms and conditions presented on any website of Bentham Science Publishers conflict with, or are inconsistent with, the terms and conditions set out in this License Agreement, you acknowledge that the terms and conditions set out in this License Agreement shall prevail.

**Bentham Science Publishers Pte. Ltd.**
80 Robinson Road #02-00
Singapore 068898
Singapore
Email: subscriptions@benthamscience.net

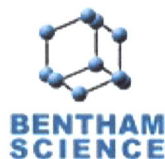

# CONTENTS

# PREFACE

This eBook series entitled, *"Frontiers in Occupational Health and Safety"* with volume title **"Introduction to Occupational Health Hazards"** is an effort to underline the significance of the safety and well-being of workers in occupational settings.

The book has 6 chapters divided into four units by various authors. Each chapter showcases a new aspect of occupational hazard.

Unit I: Introduction to Occupational Hazards

Unit II: Kinds of Diseases Induced by Various Occupations

Unit III: Occupational Hazards Associated with Various Professions

Unit IV: Previously Unrecognized Occupational Hazard

I am highly grateful to **Dr. S. M. Hadi**, Emeritus Professor, Department of Biochemistry, AMU, an accomplished scientist for keeping his promise of briefly reviewing the book and writing a 'Foreword' despite paucity of time.

I would like to express my gratitude to all the authors for bearing patience during the long time this book took to see light of the day.

**Unit I:** New Frontiers in Occupational Disease

The introductory chapter, tries to encompass the emerging and existing occupational disorders some of which were earlier unnoticed or were unborn until recently into six disease causing agents, biological, chemical, physical, ergonomic, psychosocial and accidental. Emergence of newer disorders in the aftermath of industrialization, globalization, migration, extremes of climatic conditions, recreation methods has become possible due to the advancement of science and technology. The role of various international organizations like WHO, ILO *etc.* is highlighted on pertinent issues. This book aims to deviate from traditionally discussed occupational hazards to focus on work-related hazards which evolved with advent of newer professions.

**UNIT II:** Kinds of Diseases Induced by Various Occupations

**This unit** takes two examples Neurological disorders and Cancer as subject to study kinds of occupational diseases.

**Dr. Kumar Vaibhav** a seasoned Neurotoxicologist from Department of Neurosurgery, Medical College of Georgia, Augusta University along with **Dr. Rajesh Yadav** of **Dr. HG Central** University has tried to summarize "Occupational Hazards as Neurological Disorders".

**Dr. Manzur Gattu** and **Sufia Naseem** are biochemists from JN Medical College, AMU trying to give us a holistic view of to the world of occupational cancers.

**UNIT III:** Occupational Hazards Associated with Various Professions

Medicine is the one of the ancient and noble profession. Nosocomial infections are infections acquired by hospital staff at work. Me and **Professor Shagufta Moin** along with her team from JN Medical College, AMU, has tried to give insight into the medico world of susceptibility and risks associated with medical and paramedical work. It also highlights the fact that following simple preventive measures can save lives of thousands of trained and untrained workers in health sector including doctors and nurses.

Noted Scientist Parie Curie died of Cancer. Accidents in academia are frequent in developed and developing countries. Genetically Modified Organisms (GMO), Recombinant DNA (R-DNA), Biological expression systems, transgenic and knock out animals, transgenic plants, biological waste or combination of biological and radiation waste are new age professional hazards for scientists. The hepatitis B virus is several times more contagious than HIV, a medical professional/scientist coming in contact with hepatitis B is likely to be infected without proper vaccination or other precautions. For the first time, a comprehensive chapter regarding the "awareness of biosafety issues of scientists" has been written by me in collaboration with **Professor Achla Gupta** of Mount Sinai School of Medicine for the benefit of all the students and researchers. The chapter successfully marks that following stringent precautions is essential before establishing a laboratory and while scientists are at work. Also, proper disposal procedures must be followed after the scientific task is completed to avoid any risk of infection/accident for the scientist and general public.

**UNIT IV:** Previously Unrecognized Occupational Hazard

This unit has one chapter articulating the case of previously unrecognized health hazard 'mental stress' of the workforce. Stress was an unknown term during the first half of the century bygone. Lack of proper sleep and change in biological clocks is leading to a lesser understood but almost an epidemic like disease-Stress. The last twenty years have seen the enhancement of the reported cases of stress, so is the rise in consumption of anti-depressants. The previously unrecognized occupational hazard forms a common denominator for almost all work place issues. Adequate sleep has gained significance as it tries to bring down levels of Stress. I have tried to study stress as a component of anxiety and collapse of circadian rhythm.

I would like to thank the entire team Bentham Science Publishers for being partners in production of this eBook. The people from Bentham Science Publishers who deserve special mention are, Ms. Fariya Zulfiqar, Mr. Shehzad Naqvi and Mr. Mahmood Alam.

I would like to thank Prof. S.J. Rizvi for being my mentor and guide.

Last but not the least; I would thank my parents, husband, brother and kids for generating the support system around me that keeps me steady.

**Farhana Zahir**
Prism Educational Society,
Aligarh, U.P.,
India

# FOREWORD

It is a pleasure for me to write a foreword for the book series entitled, "Frontiers in Occupational Health and safety" with volume title "Introduction to occupational health hazards" by Dr. Farhana Zahir. Much scientific literature is available on the subject; nevertheless, the contents are of topical interest in the context of the current industrial scene in the entire world. Indeed, various international organizations including WHO have issued guidelines for the safety of workforce in various industries. A healthy workforce is of vital concern for sustainable social and economic development on global, national and local levels. The classical approach to ensuring health and safety of the workforce has depended mainly on the enactment of necessary legislation and inspection of workplace. Unfortunately, in many of the third world countries, the industrial workplaces remain insecure in spite of the existence of the required legislation.

I believe that the contents of the present work are of adequate scientific value and would be of interest to both the established workers in the field as well as those who would like to have a general idea of the hazards involved in various industries. The book also contains a chapter on previously unrecognized hazards such as physical stress and mental health of the workers which should be of particular interest to the readers.

**Prof. S.M. Hadi**
Emeritus Professor
Department of Biochemistry,
Aligarh Muslim University, Aligarh,
India

# List of Contributors

**Achla Gupta**
Department of Pharmacological Sciences, Ichan School of Medicine at Mount Sinai, New York, USA

**Abdul Faiz Faizy**
Department of Biochemistry, JN Medical College, Aligarh Muslim University, Aligarh, Uttar Pradesh, India

**Farhana Zahir**
Prism Educational Society, Aligarh, U.P., India

**Kumar Vaibhav**
Department of Neurosurgery, Augusta University, 1120 15th St, Augusta 30912 (GA), Augusta, USA

**Manzoor Ahmad Gatoo**
Department of Biochemistry, JN Medical College, AMU, Aligarh, Uttar Pradesh, India

**Nasreen Noor**
Department of Obstetrics and Gynaecology, JN Medical College, Aligarh Muslim University, Aligarh, Uttar Pradesh, India

**Rajesh Singh Yadav**
Department of Criminology and Forensic Science, School of Applied Sciences, Dr. Harisingh Gour Central University, Sagar 470 003 (MP), India

**Shazia Parveen**
Department of Obstetrics and Gynaecology, JN Medical College, Aligarh Muslim University, Aligarh, Uttar Pradesh, India

**Shaziya Allarakha**
Department of Biochemistry, JN Medical College, Aligarh Muslim University, Aligarh, Uttar Pradesh, India

**Shagufta Moin**
Department of Biochemistry, JN Medical College, Aligarh Muslim University, Aligarh, Uttar Pradesh, India

**Sufia Naseem**
Department of Biochemistry, JN Medical College, AMU, Aligarh, Uttar Pradesh, India

# CHAPTER 1

# New Frontiers in Occupational Disease

## Farhana Zahir[*]

*Prism Educational Society, Aligarh, U.P., India*

**Abstract:** If a disease demonstrates frequency in a group of people of a particular occupation more than the one that takes place in general public and has a demonstrable record between a particular illness and specific work/work-related environment, it is classified as an occupational disease. The development of a new class of occupational disorders is by-product of the recent uncontrolled man-man, man-machine and man-agents' interaction. A small percentage of workers amongst the total working population of the world have access to occupational health related services, the access gets diminished if the worker is a child labour from a developing country. Moreover, the constant evolution of newer work areas and substances has led to continuous revision of list of causative agents and occupational health hazards by various agencies. "Diving medicine" is one such emerging branch of medicine dealing with specific health aspects of deep sea divers. The study of cause-effect relationship of occupational diseases will contribute towards reducing cases of work related disorders. Biological agents become causative agents through generation of bio aerosols or as routine infectious agents affecting biomedical scientists, laboratory technicians, medical and paramedical staff. The duration of exposure and varying doses (low-high) of hazardous chemical complexes are a source of a range of disorders from long term effects like neuro- behavioural dysfunction to immediate effects like burns. Some substances sensitise both airways and skin leading to respiratory and skin disorders. Similarly, the intensity and duration of exposure to the physical agents lead to an array of disorders ranging from white finger vibration, trench foot, barotrauma upto cancer. Besides exposure to biological, chemical, physical, ergonomic disease causing agents a worker is also prone to altered psychosocial agents at workplace. Violence and accidents occur at workplace. Discrimination (gender/ethnic/ migrant status), disturbed circadian rhythm, work pressure, lack of job satisfaction and social life leading to depression and anxiety have become a new normal in working class.

**Keywords:** Bacteria, Bradford Hill's Criteria, Compressed or decompressed air, Universal diagnostic criteria, Ergonomic agent, Extremes of temperature, Fungi, International Labour Organization, Needle-stick injury, Noise, Occupational diseases, Organic Dust, Parasites, Protein, Psychosocial agent, Radiation, Respiratory disorders, Skin disorders, **Sa substances (Substances causing**,

[*] **Corresponding author Farhana Zahir:** Prism Educational Society, Aligarh, U.P., India; Tel: +91 9760986931; +91 798386098; Email: farhanazahir@gmail.com

**airway sensitisation)**, Vibration, Viruses, WHO, work-related Musculoskeletal Disorders (WRMSDs).

## INTRODUCTION

The first incidence of work-related disorder was identified in 1775 in 'Chimney sweep boys'. Half of the worlds' population is worker. Occupational disorders have become widespread as a by-product of industrialization and globalization. As per the statistics given by International Labour Organization (ILO) in a single year (2000), 2 million people died, around 271 million people were injured and about 160 million people became ill as a result of occupation-related health hazards. The risk of occupational diseases increases many folds in case of accidents like Bhopal methyl isocyanide leakage or the recent japanese tsunami which led to thermal reactors' meltdown.

In early days, only industry workers or mine workers especially those working in coal mines were considered to be exposed to health hazards owing to their occupation. But now-a- days, modern concept of health has widened the scope of Occupational disorders by including all types of service trades, agriculture, health care sector and ergonomics. Newer occupations like those of biomedical scientists (*e.g.*, conducting research on deadly Ebola/Marburg virus/Zika Virus) or medical laboratory technicians (*e.g.,* performing diagnostic test of TB) create previously unrecognized occupational disorders. Unconventional health risks which come under occupational hazard are extreme climatic conditions (*e.g.*, armed forces working on high altitude/scientists working in Antarctica), long hours use of computer, Vibrations (*e.g.*, Transport vehicle) *etc.* Work-related stress due to lack of sleep, mental trauma *etc.* and violence as faced by medical staff are all other recognized occupational hazards. **The magnitude of increment in cases of work-related diseases pressurises International Labour Organization to add new substances/sources to their list after every few years.** Any disease contracted as a result of exposure to risk factors arising from work activity is termed Occupational Disease according to Occupational Safety and Health Convention, protocol 2002. For any disease to qualify as occupational disease it must demonstrate disease frequency more than general public and have a demonstrable record between a particular illness and specific work/work-related environment.

In accordance with World Health Organization reports, only 15% global workforce has access to Occupational health-related services. This becomes more complicated when 70% of world's working population live in developing countries. Further, the fact that people most vulnerable to work-related disorders come from the weakest sections of the society makes the issue more complicated.

As per the statics issued by International Labour Organization, children between the age group 5-17 comprise 352 million work force, of which 170 million work in perilous settings despite serious intervention of 130 countries making stringent child labour laws. **The physical, moral and mental fabric of child workers undergoes irreversible loss when they work in dangerous situations without proper access to basic health amenities. Many child workers acquire illness which last a lifetime.**

Occupational diseases are avoidable, if proper care is taken. Therefore, it becomes imperative to study cause-effect relationship; though, complexities of human behaviour also play a role, for instance, willingness of a worker to adapt to strict hygiene/wear a helmet or take other safety precautions. The manner in which human body interacts within a certain work environment determines its stress level. But the previous work history of the person is also a determining factor while studying his susceptibility towards disease. Body-burden of slow metabolizing substances (like chromium or lead or benzene), physical distortion (like Carpel Tunnel syndrome) acquired at an earlier work will certainly influence his chances of acquiring a malady. Gene pool, age, gender, health, race, lifestyle are other aspects which will undoubtedly manipulate one's likelihood of acquiring a disease. The source of information for such analysis primarily comes from epidemiological and scientific studies. Industrial accidents like Chernobyl also contribute vast amount of data.

There are three kinds of Interactions (Fig. **1**) a person is supposed to experience during his/her working year. They are man-man (biological interaction), man-machine (physical interaction), man-work agents (chemical interaction).

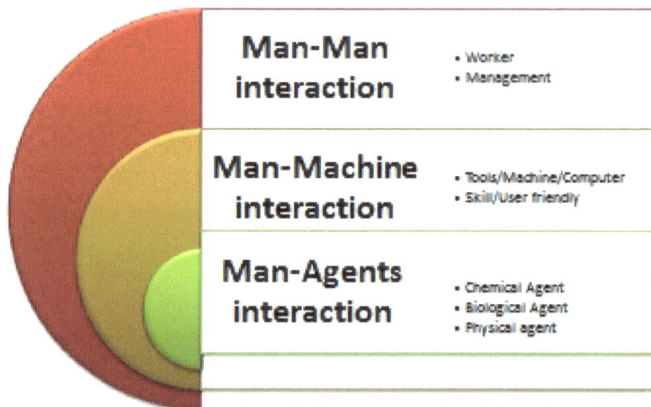

**Fig. (1).** The web of interactions.

## Man-Man Interactions (Biological Interaction)

The interaction between workers and management or amongst the workers must remain smooth under ideal conditions. Man-man interactions, whenever get adverse at work place, may lead to anxiety and depression which in turn, may be a cause of violence/harassment/abuse or in extreme cases may take the magnitude of murder or suicide or even both.

## Man-Machine Interaction (Physical Interaction)

The interaction of a man with tools or introduction of new tools or machines is very important. For instance, introduction of computers in every field like, designing, education, transport, construction, and diagnostics in the last few decades has a huge impact on workforce and **work ethics**. It also depends on age and skill level of the worker. The user-friendly design of the machine is important besides the ergonomic design of the visual display unit at workplace. Man-machine interactions in their subtlest form may lead to mild emotional strain or musculoskeletal disorder while in extreme cases any fault in the machinery/ improper use of the equipment/lack of safety measures/human error may result in ghastly accidents leading to lifelong disability or death in worst cases.

## Man-Work Agents Interaction (Chemical Interaction)

The interaction of workers with agents of work like use of toxic chemicals (**Chemical agent**) or handling infectious materials (**Biological agents**) or extremes of temperature or constant vibrations (**Physical agents**) may lead to compromised health of the worker or may lead to permanent disability or may even prove to be fatal.

## Universal Diagnostic Criteria for Identification of Occupational Diseases

The duration of exposure, uniformity and specificity serve as universal diagnostic criteria (Fig. **2**) for identification of occupational disease. In order to qualify as occupational disease besides duration of exposure, uniformity and specificity, preliminary interventional studies must support the occupational disease.

### *Duration of Exposure*

The longer the duration of exposure the greater the impact, hence, stronger is the likelihood for the development of the disease.

### *Uniformity*

There should be coherence in results/reports from various laboratories regarding the disease. All epidemiological and animal studies must demonstrate cause and effect relationship.

## *Specificity*

Exposure to a definite risk factor results in a noticeably defined pattern of ailment.

## *Interventional Studies*

A primary preventive trial may suggest removal of a specific risk factor or hazard from a particular work environment to remove incidence of a specific disease.

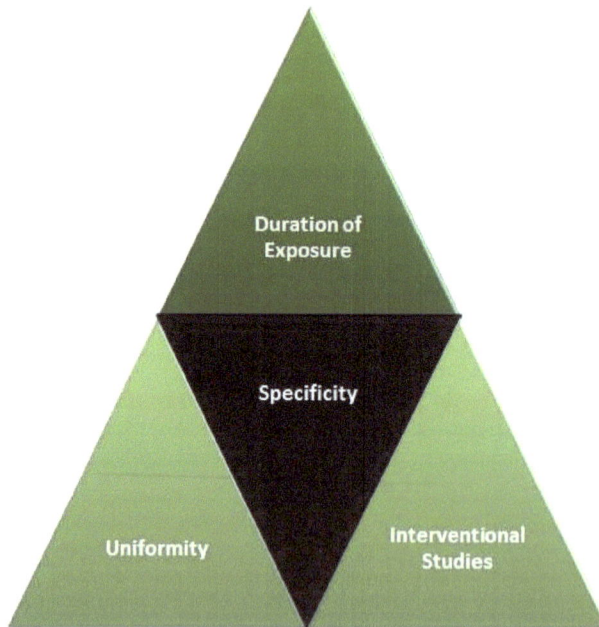

**Fig. (2).** Universal Diagnostic Criteria.

## Bradford Hill's Criteria

In 1965, Sir Austin Bradford Hill proposed a criteria using cause-effect in identification of disease. It is widely used by epidemiologists even today after 53 years since it was first published; despite a lot of debate over its absoluteness. The nine point criteria, famously known as **Hill's Criteria** include Strength, Consistency, Specificity, Temporality, Biological gradient, Plausibility, Coherence, Experiment and Analogy for identification of disease. It was using this approach he demonstrated the relationship between cigarette smoking and lung cancer. As occupational diseases are studied in a live setting there is an intrinsic chance of error which must be eliminated during statistical analysis before making final conclusion while using Hill's Criteria. The anticipated types of errors are random, systematic and logical.

## Broad Classification of Occupational Diseases

The Occupational diseases can be broadly classified according to disease causing agents. Thus, there are following six classes of diseases (Fig.**3**).

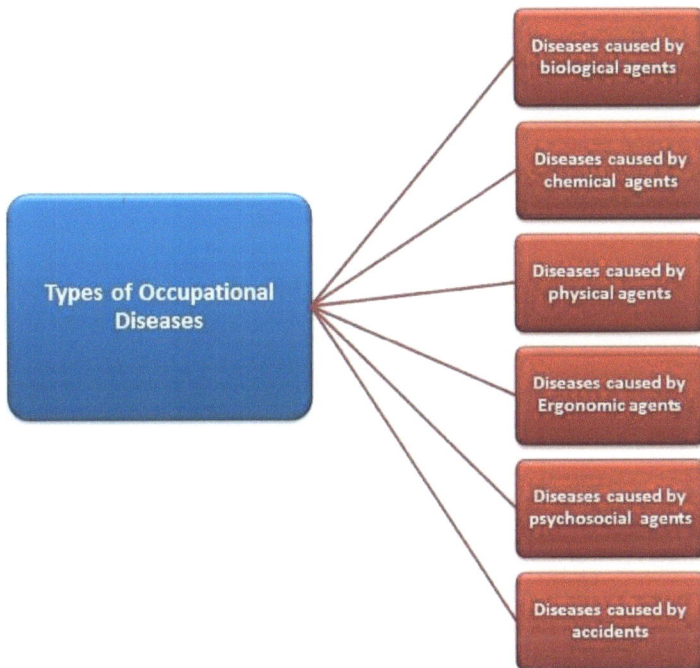

**Fig. (3).** Broad Classification of Occupational Diseases.

1. Disease caused by Biological agent.
2. Disease caused by Chemical agent.
3. Disease caused by Physical agent.
4. Disease caused by Ergonomic agent.
5. Disease caused by Psychosocial agent.
6. Disease caused by Accidents.

## Occupational Diseases caused by Biological Agent

Bacteria, Fungi, Viruses, Parasites and Proteins can act as disease causing biological agents (Fig. **4**). There are two ways by which biological agents act as occupational hazard. The first way is generation of bio aerosols and second is as the routine infectious agent. Any particulate matter of organic origin is defined as bioaerosol [1]. Pollen grains, bedding material, manure, molds, high molecular polymers released by bacteria and fungi (termed endotoxin or beta glucans, respectively), low molecular polymers released by fungi called mycotoxins, volatile organic compounds *etc.* may form bioaerosol. Biological agents of disease are elaborately discussed in chapters **3, 4 & 5.**

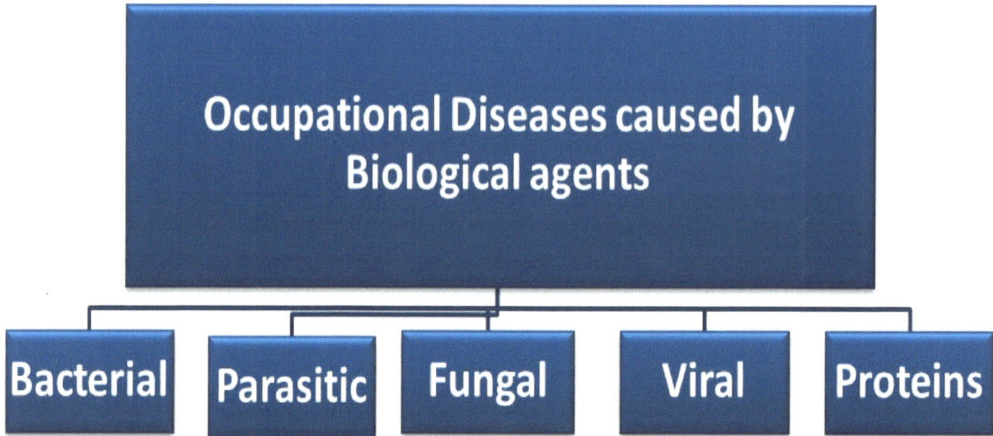

**Occupational Diseases caused by Biological agents**

| Bacterial | Parasitic | Fungal | Viral | Proteins |

**Fig. (4).** Broad classification of Occupational Diseases caused by Biological agents.

## *Bacterial Infections*

Methicillin-resistant *Staphylococcus aureus* (MRSA) is a bacterial strain reported in hospital settings since 1960.It causes a spectrum of diseases related to soft tissue and skin rashes, abscesses *etc.* As *Staphylococcus aureus* is a drug resistant bacterium, it is a threat to hospital staff like doctors, nurses and students [2]. Work-related Sarcoidosis is a multiorgan granulomatous disease with presumably mouldy or mycobacterium indoor office or nano particle exposure as has emerged from World Trade Centre office respondents [3]. Legionellosis is a pneumonia like infection is caused due to a bacterium (*L. pneumophilal*) by exposure to aerosol generated by water. Workers of telephone manholes [4], glass processing industry [5] and non-industrial working environment [6] like wastewater treatment plants, cooling towers, and humidifiers are well known as the patients for disease. Multi drug resistant gram negative enteric pathogens (GNEP) **have also recently emerged as a problem to animal husbandry. Nosocomial Infections or hospital acquired infections** are discussed in detail in chapter **4**. But development of Carbapenem-resistant Enterobacteriacae like New Delhi metallo-β-lactamase (NDM-1) has become a major cause of public health concern worldwide due to the development of drug resistant mutants.

## Ectoparasitic Infections

Insects like fleas, sand flies and ticks act as vectors to pathogens like virus, bacteria or protozoa to cats and dogs. They are therefore, considered as potential health threat to their care givers and veterinary experts. Canine Vector-borne diseases (CVBD) and Feline Vector-borne diseases (FVBD)are terms used to describe the diseases transmitted through dogs and cats, respectively. The prime diseases under CVBD are rickettsiosis, tick borreliosis and canine leishmaniasis [7]. Ticks also pose serious health threat [8] to landscape developers and gardeners *etc.* particularly in Europe. Other pathogens spread by ticks include *Anaplasma phagocytophilum*, *Borrelia burgdorferi*, and *Ehrlichia canis*. Mosquitoes spread microfilariae of *Dirofilaria immitis* in dogs besides famously spreading malarial parasite.

## Fungal Infections

Mycotoxins represent the only established non-viral occupational carcinogens [11]. Pulmonary cancers are reported in workers exposed to aflatoxin in industrial settings [12]. Denmark has previous incidences of liver cancer to workers during exposures to aflatoxin during farm work [13].

*Stachybotrys chartarum* is cellulolytic and causes soft rot of wood. It is usually found associated with damp straw and wall paper. It was first reported from wall paper in the city of Prague, the Czech Republic. Dampness attracts *Stachybotrys chartarum,* the most common allergenic fungi found indoors in offices, school, homes [14] and farms in countries like USA, Canada, Russia, Hungary, Bosnia Herzegovinia,Germany, France, North and south Africa. Air-borne fungi are found in very high concentrations of office archives. The four common fungi reported are *Cladosporium* sp., *Aspergillus* sp., *Penicillium* sp., *Stachybotrys chartarum*. Moulds belonging to these genera are also reported during grain loading and unloading. They are causative agents of farmer's lung disease [15]. Dairy farmers are also prone to infection from *Stachybotrys chartarum* as the fungus has been found in dairy cattle shed [11]. Early reports suggest severe lung infection on exposure while handling straw. A recent report states presence of *Stachybotrys chartarum* chemotype in dried culinary herbs [16]. This indicates occupational exposure of farm workers and hospital staff to the fungus. Today, the infection has been controlled using building technology to control dampness.

Waste water treatment plants (**WWTP**) all over Europe have reported presence of filamentous fungi in the air and water samples from their sites. In a study of two Portuguese WWTP, *Penicillium* sp. was the most frequently isolated fungal genus (58.9%), followed by *Aspergillus* sp. (21.2%) and *Acremonium* sp. (8.2%), in the total underground area [17]. In a partially underground plant, *Penicillium* sp.

(39.5%) was also the most frequently isolated, followed by *Aspergillus* sp. (38.7%) and *Acremonium* sp. (9.7%). Therefore, the workers of these WWTPs are at occupational risk to fungal infections.

A Podiatrist is also exposed to bioaerosols loaded with fungus and yeast causing respiratory distress [18].

### Algal Infections

The toxins produced by algae adversely affect humans, aquatic animals and ecosystems.

### Viral Infections

Healthcare workers, research staff particularly those who are pregnant are high risk populations for human immunodeficiency virus, hepatitis B virus, hepatitis C virus, varicella-zoster virus, herpes simplex virus, human parvovirus B19, cytomegalovirus, rubella, measles, enteroviruses, mumps and influenza. In a comparative review, 84% laboratory infections were through aerosols including lymphocyctic choriomeningitis virus infections, hantavirus and coxsackievirus infections while droplet and mucocutaneous were leading transmission modes for **Severe acute respiratory syndrome (SARS)** and **influenza B,** respectively [9]. The deadly SARS infection is caused by Coronavirus. The same study found 92% blood borne viral infections to be contracted while working in hospitals.

Encephalitis in animal farmers is caused by Nipah virus in pigs and Hendra virus in horses while Haemorrhagic fever with renal syndrome (HFRS) or pulmonary syndrome (HPS) in farmers and laboratory workers is caused by Hantavirus by infecting field rodents [10].

### Protein Diseases

Prions are responsible for zoonotic variant of Creutzfeldt-Jakob disease in agricultural and laboratory workers. Meat and bone meal is a well-known source for prion disease. Meat processing industry caters packed meat to millions. Its by-product bone meal and discarded meat is used in making fertilizers, animal feed and as alternative fuel. Thousands of workers are employed in meat industry or those using animal feed or fertilizer made from meat and bone meal besides those employed in storehouses and transportation or those who work in power stations using fuel made from infected meat. All these workers are at great risk of exposure to prions which lead to a series of neurodegenerative diseases. Though certain procedures are used to minimize prions, none of them are foolproof [19].

**Occupational pollinosis** has been recorded in professional gardeners or green house workers rearing ornamental flowers like chrysanthemum or fruits like strawberries or to paddy farmers.

## Occupational Diseases Caused by Chemical Agents

There is a range of chemical substances (Fig. **5**) from pure elements to their oxides, sulphites, carbonates or radioisotopes which are either found naturally or are produced artificially like polymers. Acrylamides, solvents, organophosphate compounds like insecticides, organic, halogenous compounds and various gases are few high risk chemicals to which workers are exposed.

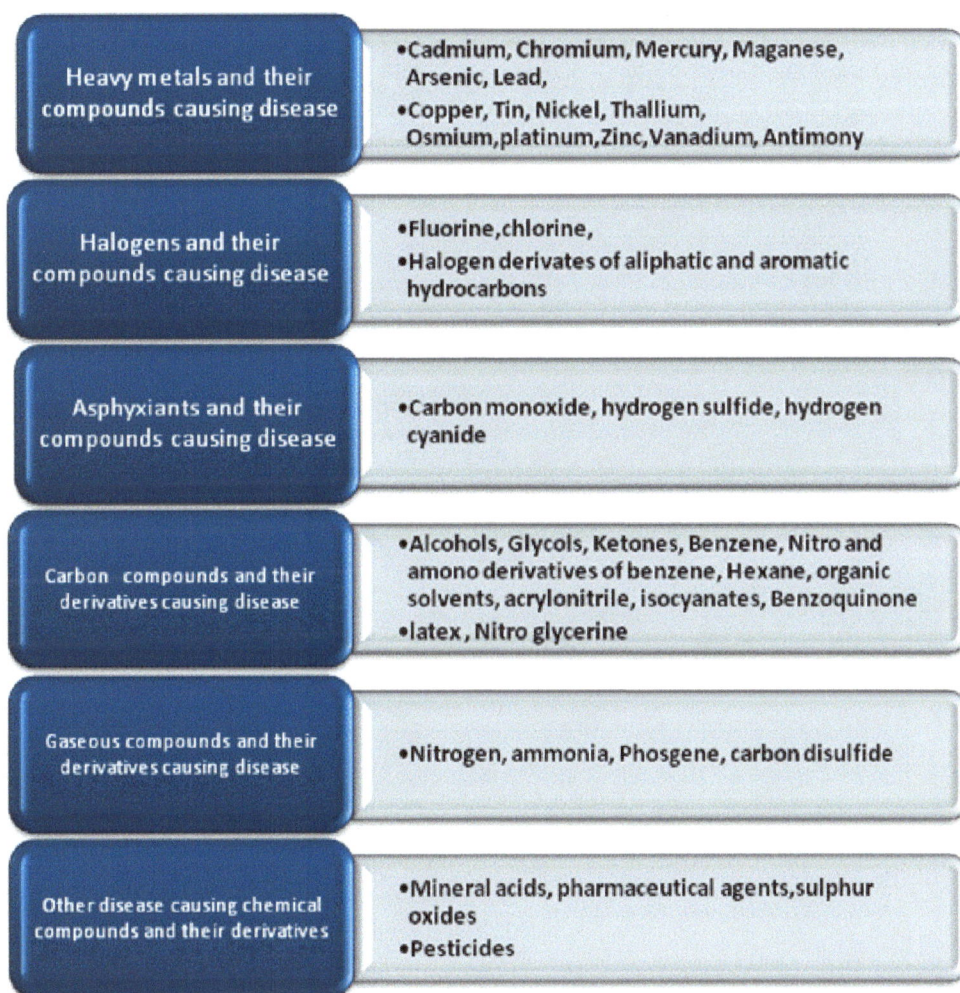

| | |
|---|---|
| Heavy metals and their compounds causing disease | • Cadmium, Chromium, Mercury, Maganese, Arsenic, Lead, <br> • Copper, Tin, Nickel, Thallium, Osmium, platinum, Zinc, Vanadium, Antimony |
| Halogens and their compounds causing disease | • Fluorine, chlorine, <br> • Halogen derivates of aliphatic and aromatic hydrocarbons |
| Asphyxiants and their compounds causing disease | • Carbon monoxide, hydrogen sulfide, hydrogen cyanide |
| Carbon compounds and their derivatives causing disease | • Alcohols, Glycols, Ketones, Benzene, Nitro and amono derivatives of benzene, Hexane, organic solvents, acrylonitrile, isocyanates, Benzoquinone <br> • latex, Nitro glycerine |
| Gaseous compounds and their derivatives causing disease | • Nitrogen, ammonia, Phosgene, carbon disulfide |
| Other disease causing chemical compounds and their derivatives | • Mineral acids, pharmaceutical agents, sulphur oxides <br> • Pesticides |

**Fig. (5).** Indicative list of various chemicals and their derivatives either during manufacturing process or during use.

The workers might be exposed to a level well below the threshold value. But, continuous exposure to low doses of chemical compounds/heavy metals over a period of time has become a source of concern [20].

Heavy metals like lead, mercury, chromium, arsenic, cadmium become sources of exposure when they are extracted from earth by mining. Heavy metals listed in Fig. (**6**) have numerous industrial, scientific and medicinal applications ranging from Gold mining which uses mercury amalgam, use of lead and arsenic in manufacture of glass and paints, control of nuclear fission by cadmium rods, arsenic compound Lewisite has been used as chemical weapon. The list given below indicates a few uses of heavy metals which expose the manufacturers, people like painters who actually use the product carrying the toxic compounds. Long term exposure to inorganic lead leads to peripheral neuropathy [21]. Neurobehavioral test scores have demonstrated that long term occupational lead exposure may lead to progressive decline in cognitive functions [22]. **The literature has vast data on the toxicity of chemical agents. The topic is vast enough to be covered as a separate book.**

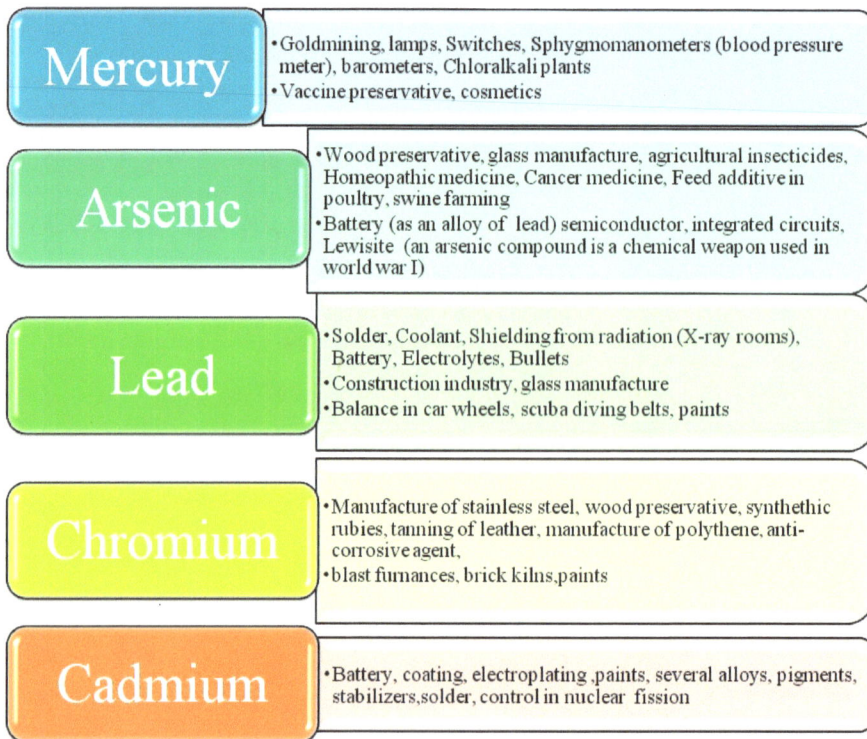

| Mercury | • Goldmining, lamps, Switches, Sphygmomanometers (blood pressure meter), barometers, Chloralkali plants<br>• Vaccine preservative, cosmetics |
|---------|---------------------------------------------------------------------------------------------------|
| Arsenic | • Wood preservative, glass manufacture, agricultural insecticides, Homeopathic medicine, Cancer medicine, Feed additive in poultry, swine farming<br>• Battery (as an alloy of lead) semiconductor, integrated circuits, Lewisite (an arsenic compound is a chemical weapon used in world war I) |
| Lead | • Solder, Coolant, Shielding from radiation (X-ray rooms), Battery, Electrolytes, Bullets<br>• Construction industry, glass manufacture<br>• Balance in car wheels, scuba diving belts, paints |
| Chromium | • Manufacture of stainless steel, wood preservative, synthethic rubies, tanning of leather, manufacture of polythene, anti-corrosive agent,<br>• blast furnances, brick kilns, paints |
| Cadmium | • Battery, coating, electroplating, paints, several alloys, pigments, stabilizers, solder, control in nuclear fission |

**Fig. (6).** Indicative list of sources of exposure to Heavy metals either during manufacturing process or during use.

The malfunctioning of haematopoietic system, heart, thyroid, allergies, neurotoxicity are previously well known effects of cobalt. Tinnitus, deafness, vertigo, visual changes, optic atrophy, tremor bilateral optic atrophy and retinopathy, bilateral nerve deafness, sensory-motor polyneuropathy and peripheral neuropathy are other occupational risks of Cobalt [23]. Besides, chemical burns are a routine while working with hazardous chemicals. For instance, Hydroflouric acid (HF) burns are reported at neck, head and upper extremities and are regular in both male and female workers in the western Zhejiang province of China as reported by a 10-year epidemiological study [24]. Moreover, electrolyte balance of Calcium and Magnesium was also disturbed in such workers [24]. Inhalation injury, ocular burns and digestive tract injury are accompanying injuries in chemical burns.

## Occupational Diseases Caused by Physical Agents

Occupational diseases caused by exposure to physical agents arising from work activities are broadly listed in Fig. (**7**). The physical agents like noise, vibrations, temperature extremes, radiations *etc.* contribute to a lot of distress. Jobs which require high physical exertion like flight attendants and teachers also risk their pregnancy.

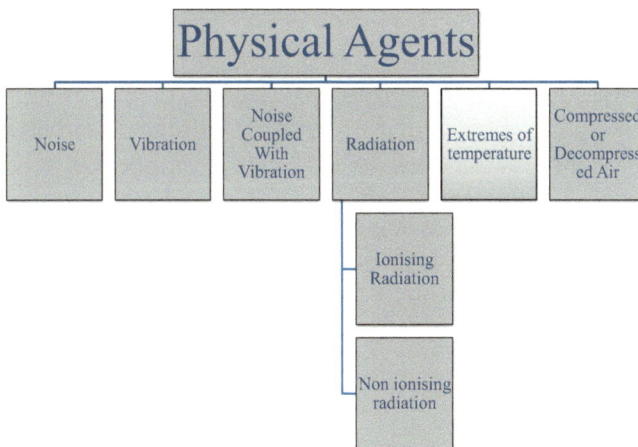

**Fig. (7).** Broad category of disease causing physical agents.

## *Noise*

It is a well-recognized occupational hazard. Occupational noise exposure in restaurants [25] and factories may lead to temporary or permanent hearing loss. Noise induced hearing loss depends on duration of exposure and decibels. A dose response relationship has been found between in-ear occupational noise exposure and hearing loss amongst industrial workers [26]. It affects all age groups. There are a number of non-auditory health effects [27] associated with noise like headache, annoyance, fatigue, sleep disturbance contributing to noise-stress related burn out. It has been reported that noise stress related burnout in hospital staff leads to low well-being and poor performance [28]. High noise leads to speech intelligibility thus the misunderstandings at times lead to medical errors. The other non-auditory impact of noise is hypertension leading to cardiovascular disease [29]. Occupational noise annoyance has been linked to depression and suicidal tendency in a nationwide study in Korea [30].

## Noise Coupled with Vibration

The prevalence of hypertension and obliterating endarteritis was found statistically higher in professionals who were exposed to noise and vibrations both [31]. Studies have linked increased risk of noise induced hearing loss with white finger vibration in occupational settings [32].

## Vibration Stress

Various disorders of bones, blood vessels, nerves, joints, muscles or connective tissue of hand and fore arm are due to use of vibrating tools leading to a syndrome called **Vibration induced white finger (VWF).** There is a clear relationship between level of vibration, duration of exposure and prevalence of vibration induced white finger [33]. Vibration stress have been found to have a direct dose response relationship in development of musculoskeletal disorders of neck and upper limb in forestry workers exposed to hand-arm vibration [34].

According to a study, about 30% working population amounting to 4.5 million people of Czech Republic suffers from musculoskeletal disorders owing to their occupations which involve vibrations (2.6%), physical work (16%) and wrong posture (16%) [35]. Continuous vibrations may lead to neuropathy, for which there is no cure except some ergonomic measures [36].

## Hazards from Radiation

In order to study radiation hazards in detail a separate chapter is required. Nuclear radiation risks from power plants are well known. It is estimated that exposure to medical radiation has been increased 600% due to use of imaging tools like CT scan and intervention radiology [37]. Doctors performing interventional radiology without any preventive measure may receive doses leading to lens opacity [38]. In a survey on US flight attendants, it was found that 0.1 mGy cosmic exposures maybe associated with miscarriage [39]. Maternal occupational exposure to ionizing radiation may cause major structural birth defects [40]. A study of outdoor workers working in local government Organizations in Colorado demonstrated a need for safety gear hat, eye, overall clothing to reduce exposure to sun radiation as a measure to reduce skin cancer risk [41].

## *Brief Guidelines for Prevention of Occupational Radiation Injury*

Regulation of protection from radiation at medical or industrial sector should be strictly followed in order to minimize the occupational exposure (Fig. **8**).

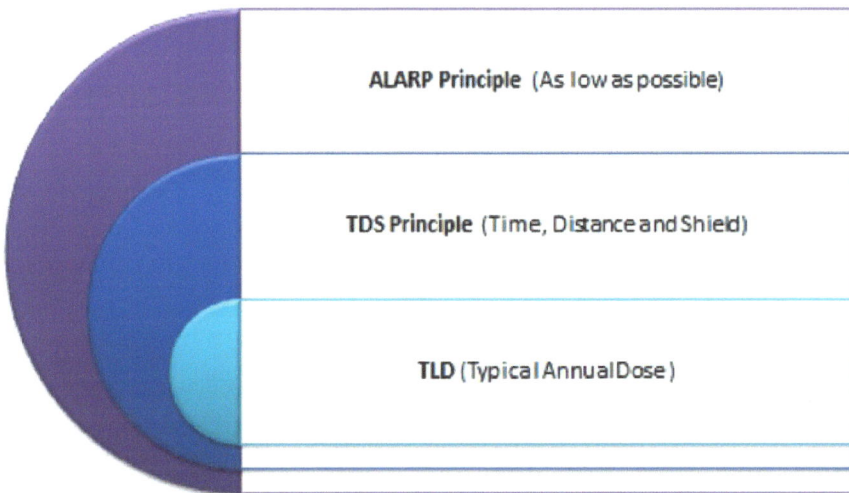

ALARP Principle (As low as possible)

TDS Principle (Time, Distance and Shield)

TLD (Typical Annual Dose)

**Fig. (8).** Basic rules to prevent radiation.

a. The facility using radioactive material is advised to keep 'radiation as low as reasonably achievable' (**ALARA**) through strict monitoring of the facility (through recent dosimetry techniques) and by establishing guidelines and their strict enforcement through inspection.
   The controlled areas should have minimum prescribed dose levels and adequate display of warning signs. The authorities are encouraged to optimise procedure routinely so as to expose the workers to the lowest possible radiation.
b. The golden rule for workers and organizations is to strictly abide by **TDS principle** (Time, Distance and Shield). The TLD (typical annual dose) for people working on high energy machines is 0.2mSv. Lead shields and doors are erected to minimise radiation.
c. For low energy radiation like x-rays and gamma rays, lead aprons are recommended while for facilities with high energy radiation like neutron, fixed

dose detectors are required.
d. The International Commission for Radiological Protection is an independent non-government organization which issues periodically updated advisories, for instance **IRCP 118** which includes information on radiation risk of tissues known as *deterministic effects.*
**Asian Pacific Society for Interventional Cardiology** and **Society for Cardiovascular Angiography and Interventions** have laid down strict guidelines to reduce radiation exposure to physicians and allied staff to reduce percutaneous coronary intervention electrophysiology procedure like minimising fluoroscopy time and number of acquired images. Routine medical examination is done for the analysis of radiation induced damage for biomarkers of cancer.
e. Immediate detection of leakage at source.

### Hazards from Extremes of Temperature

Extremes of temperature either too hot or too cold are likely to disturb the routine functioning of the body, thus reducing work productivity. Thermal extremes may be experienced during indoor or outdoor work, or a combination of both which might be aggravated by protective clothing or lack of proper sanitation facilities. It is noteworthy that even developed economies lack sufficient guidelines for imposed heat or cold at workplace or solar ultraviolet (UV) radiation.

Every year a growing number of people working in extremely hot conditions die due to heat wave which is brought about by rising temperatures. The climate change is affecting the world economy slowly, particularly low and medium income countries in Asian and African regions, where a substantial amount of work force resides with bare minimum safety measures. Manual workers who are exposed to extreme heat or work in hot environments may be at risk of heat stress, especially those in low-middle income countries in tropical regions. At risk workers include farmers, construction workers, fire-fighters, miners, soldiers, and manufacturing workers working around process-generated heat [42]. Iron and steel foundries, brick kilns and ceramic industry are places of extreme heat exposure due to nature of work.

At temperatures around 45° C especially when hot wind called Loo blows in parts of India, a large number of people mainly construction workers or agricultural labourers die suddenly due to dehydration. The climatic conditions in tropical and sub-tropical parts of the world are currently too hot leading to loss of 15-20% annual work hours, this is expected to double by 2050 at the current pace of climate change [43]. Exposure to heat disturbs the homeostasis of body water leading to electrolyte imbalance, alteration in core temperature resulting in the development of heat cramp, heat syncope, exhaustion and stroke. Commonly coexisting risks are humidity, windlessness, infrared radiation, physical exertion, continuous work, chemical protective clothing, and lack of acclimatization [44]. The heatstroke can at times cause irreversible damage to heart, lungs, kidney and liver. Occupational burns, wounds, lacerations, and amputations as well as heat illnesses were found to be significantly associated with rise in heat in a study on workers in Adelaide, South Australia [45]. Likewise, accidents with moving objects, contact with chemicals, and injuries related to environmental factors elevated significantly during heatwaves, especially among middle-aged and older male workers [42]. A significant Persian Gulf report concludes that there is high probability of cardiac strain in obese workers in hot and humid weather [46]. Young males particularly those engaged in heavy physical work are at risk of injury on hot days and wider range of worker subgroups are vulnerable for injury following a warm night [47]. It is well known that exposure to extremes of temperature affects cognitive and motor functions.

Heat at workplace coupled with noise and high workload was found to induce Temporary Threshold Shift (TTS) in auditory capacity [48]. Electrical and chemical burns are most devastating cause of mortality at work place. Severe burns result in costly medical expenses, permanent disabilities or psychological problems or both.

Professionals of extreme sports, military, transport, public health, construction, agriculture and fisheries are exposed to extreme cold or extreme cold accompanying windy or wet or both conditions. They suffer from a range of disorders due to constriction of blood vessels and reduced metabolism depending on duration of exposure and accompanying conditions. Alcohol consumption aggravates the symptoms [44]. Occupational exposure to cold and repetitive work may lead to musculoskeletal problems [49]. Low back, knee and shoulder pain have been observed in cold store employees. Occupational exposure to cold environment for a single year alters lung function by significantly limiting airflow [50]. A study in USA shows that injuries like slips& falls have been reported to increase with falling temperature in mining industry [51]. Continuous daily exposure to cold, poor ventilation and dampness by workers of frozen food factories or cold storage may lead to back and muscle pain, respiratory symptoms, episodic finger symptoms, and cardiovascular symptoms. This is supported by a survey of frozen food processing workers in eastern Thailand [52]. A recent study shows a directly proportional correlation between increased injury and increased daily maximum temperature [48]. Extreme cold and wet conditions lead to various type of cold injuries (Fig. **9**) ranging from hypothermia to trench foot.

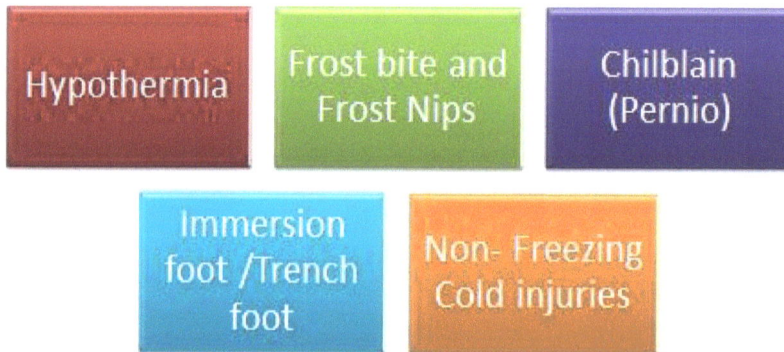

**Fig. (9).** Various types of cold injuries.

## *Hypothermia*

It is defined as decrease in core body temperature below 95°F (35°C) up to 90°F.

## *Non-Freezing Cold injuries*

These types of injuries are seen in people who work in extremely cold conditions close to freezing point for long durations [53].

## *Frost bite and Frost Nips*

Frostbite is actual freezing of tissues when body is exposed to extreme cold and sweating around -2°C for short duration (minutes to hours) while frost nip is mild originator of frostbite. Diabetes, depression, stroke and cardiac insufficiency enhances the chances of frostbite [54]. Freon gas is maintained at -41°C for use in refrigeration and air conditioning. It causes frostbite in accidental cases [55].

## *Chilblain (Pernio)*

When exposure to cold conditions occurs between 0°C to 16°C for hours and days chilblain occurs. It is exaggerated inflammatory response resulting in constriction of blood vessels and oedema [56]. It may or may not be accompanied by frostbite/frostnip. It usually affects hands and feet when a sports person wears wet clothes and moist foot-wears at very cold temperature.

## *Immersion Foot/Trench Foot*

Immersion foot /Trench foot is a condition caused by prolonged exposure to cold (0-18 ° C) and dampness for hours and days affecting nerves and blood vessels [56].

## *Hazards from Compressed or Decompressed Air*

Deep sea diving is done on an increasing scale for adventure sport and professional work like underwater archaeology, navy, exploration for marine life, oil and natural gas *etc.* According to an estimate there are seven million divers in the world and 300,000 in Korea alone [57]. Some reports consider barotrauma, decompression sickness, toxic effects of diving gases *etc.* serious and specialized enough to be considered as a separate branch of medicine. "**Diving medicine**" is a branch of medicine dealing with specific health aspects of deep sea divers.

*Barotraumas*: They are disorders of the ear and paranasal sinuses due to barometric pressure change. Barotraumas of middle and internal ear are seen in deep sea divers [58].

## Occupational Diseases caused by Ergonomic Agents

Some Prominent musculoskeletal disorders are known as occupational risks. Musculoskeletal problems have long been associated with repetitive work or forceful use of certain group of muscles (Fig. **10**). Careful examination of symptoms, diagnostic tests and work history can help a physician distinguish an occupational musculoskeletal disorder from other musculoskeletal disorders. Despite rest, application of hot or cold packs and use of anti-inflammatory drugs such injuries take years to resolve; active changes at workplace may help the patient [59].

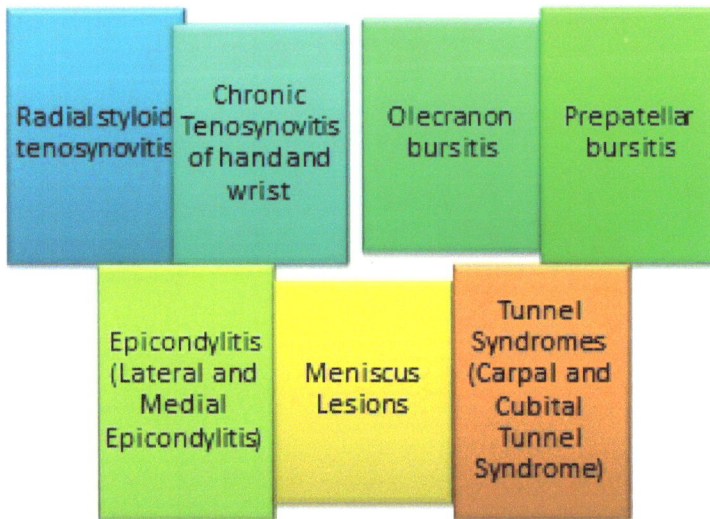

**Fig. (10).** Some prominent musculoskeletal disorders as an occupational risk.

## Work Related Musculoskeletal Disorders (WRMSDs)

They are given specialized attention these days as they cost a lot to the employer (Fig. **11**) [in terms of work quality and days/number of absent workers] and employee [in terms of reduced work days, cost of treatment and persistent pain]. Quite a lot of rehabilitation centres like RECOUP, India have started to help people with specialized requirements. High prevalence of musculoskeletal symptoms has been among employees of Iranian petrochemical industries [60]. Vibration stress has been found to have a direct dose response relationship in development of musculoskeletal disorders of neck and upper limb in forestry workers exposed to hand-arm vibration [34]. Aside, from biological hazards, dentists continue to suffer a high prevalence of musculoskeletal disorders (MSD), especially of the back, neck and shoulders.

| Musculoskeletal Disorder | • Associated Profession |
|---|---|
| De Quervain Tensosynovitis | • Opthalmologist |
| Chronic Tensosynovitis (Hand and knee) | • Housewife |
| Olecranon bursitis (or Students elbow) | • Students, Plumbers and Miners |
| Prepatellar bursitis (or Housemaid's knee) | • Carpet and Brick layers. |
| Lateral Epicondylitis (or tennis elbow) | • Automobile workers |
| Medial Epicondylitis (or golfers' elbow) | • Coal miners, Golfers |
| Cubital Tunnel Syndrome | • White Collar jobs like Computer use |
| Carpal Tunnel Syndrome | • White Collar jobs like Computer use |
| Hand arm Vibration | • Forestry Workers |

**Fig. (11).** Musculoskeletal problems associated with particular profession.

## <u>De Quervain Tensosynovitis</u>

The forceful overuse of thumb musculature leads to pain in radial aspect of wrist. The condition is called De Quervain Tensosynovitis or Radial Styloid Tenosynovitis for example, repetitive intravitreal injections triggered De Quervain Tensosynovitis in an Opthalmologist [61]. Musculoskeletal pain is very common amongst non-physician health workers who usually participate in interventional procedures.

## *Chronic Tensosynovitis (Hand and Knee)*

Chronic Tensosynovitis of **wrist** occurs due to overuse of Abductor Pollicis Longus and Extensor Pollicis Brevis tendon mostly in housewives.

Chronic Tensosynovitis of knee occurs due to forceful use of Flexor Halluces Longus tendon mostly in ballet dancers and soccer players.

## *Olecranon Bursitis*

It is also known as Students elbow. It is the inflammation of Olecranon Bursa at the back of the elbow. It is found to be associated with Students, Plumbers and Miners.

## *Prepatellar Bursitis*

It is the inflammation of Bursa at the knee. It is found to be associated with carpet and brick layers. It is also known as Housemaid's knee.

## *Epicondylitis*

It is a soft tissue injury of the elbow. There are two distinct types -lateral epicondylitis and Medial epicondylitis. Lateral  epicondylitis (also known as tennis elbow) is caused by overuse of extensor Carpi Radialis (usually found in automobile workers) while Medial Epicondylitis (also known as golfers' elbow) is caused by injury in median elbow region of Superficialis Flexor Digitorum (found in coal miners).

## *Tunnel Syndromes*

Tunnel Syndrome and Carpal Tunnel syndrome are both white collar syndromes related to upper extremity disorders of the Musculoskeletal System *e.g.*, computer professionals. Cubital Tunnel Syndrome is ulnar neuropathy due to repetitive nerve injury. Carpal Tunnel syndrome is included in European list of occupational diseases. In Germany, a physician who diagnoses Carpal tunnel syndrome is required to report the case to German Social Accident Assurance [62].

## *Meniscus Lesions*

Meniscus is a crescent shaped thick cartilaginous tissue attached to tibia, it cushions the knee from shock injury. **Meniscus tear**  may occur due to sudden twisting/flexing of knee or slowly as the cartilage loses its elasticity. For instance, excessive load on meniscus during military/sports training or sitting for long hours in squat position by coal miners might lead to tear in meniscus.

## *Some Suggested Measures to Combat Work Related Musculoskeletal Disorders (WRMSDS)*

A. Dimensions of the tools should be according to the size of the potential worker. One size fits all may not work. Women may have different comfort level for the same set of tools.
B. Total number of work hours and total force exerted on a particular joint while holding a tool in a position repetitively may be reduced to save occupational muscle injury.
C. Worker rotation.
D. Stress coupled with force, repetition and vibration is also contributing factors towards WRMSDs.

## Occupational Diseases caused by Psychosocial Agents

Today, life is viewed as a race; every single professional wants to win. But everyone can't win all the time; gradually, the pressure to perform and deliver reaches medical proportions. The **stress** it gives leads to **anxiety** and finally **depression** sets in (Fig. **12**). **Insomnia i**s being considered as a marker for mental health. A recent case control study revealed that Canadian workers' prolonged continued stress at workplace leads to cancer in 5 out of 11 cases [63]. **Malodour** at workplace due to environmental pollution leads to discomfort particularly in patients of post-traumatic stress [64].

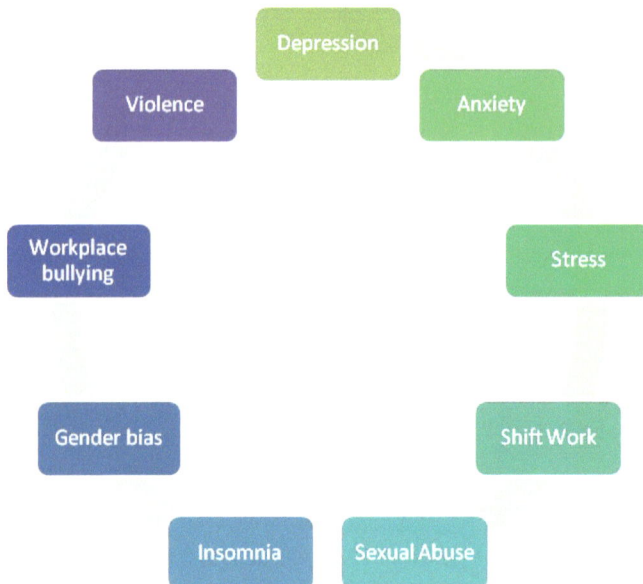

**Fig. (12).** Various Psychosocial agents at workplace.

**Violence against medical staff** particularly physicians is common. In developing countries like India, both physical and verbal violence has been reported particularly at night, mostly patients or their relatives are perpetrators [65]. **Workplace bullying** is another common problem predominant in nursing staff.

Gender bias is common which pressurizes women at work. There are thousands of reported and unreported incidences about sexual abuse at work place. Ethnic and migrant status of worker is another leading cause of discrimination.

Nursing, medical and paramedical staff, commercial vehicle drivers, airport and railway staff, hospitality industry workers, police and security agencies **work in shifts** to impart us a secure life. But long work hours coupled with irregular shift lead to fatigue disturbing circadian rhythm, sleep quantity and quality which in turn lead to accidents and injuries, deterioration in the quality of work [66].

There is growing awareness of workers' mental health issues. Lack of job satisfaction, work overload, lack of social life due to work pressure might lead to suicidal tendencies among workers. Change in work stressors is now viewed as a preventive measure to reduce suicidal tendencies. Organizations are being advised to consider providing health support to their workers as productivity and welfare of workers are inter-related [67]. A detailed discussion of work related stress can be seen in Chapter **6**.

## Occupational Diseases caused by Accidents

Each year numerous reported and unreported accidents occur at workplace both in organized and unorganized sectors (Fig. **13**). Some accidents impart lifelong disability while some are fatal. Commercial fishing has highest exposure to injury and accidental death than any other occupation.

Slips, trips, falls from ropes and ladders or due to walking-hazards on work surface are well known. Injury and mortality over a span of fifty years from 1950-2000demonstrated an elevated cohort in a Nickel refinery in Ontario, Canada [68]. Musculoskeletal disorders and fall injuries are common in household waste collectors, particularly in those with 50 years of age and above [69]. Recently, OSHA (Occupational Safety and Health Administration) has revised rules for fall protection system criteria which include design, performance and construction standards.

Industrial fires, explosions or spills of hazardous and extremely hazardous chemicals expose workers and at times residents in the adjoining areas to the toxicant and at times a lethal cocktail of accidentally mixed chemicals. For instance, accidental release of Methyl isocyanide led to the famous Bhopal Gas tragedy which immediately killed around 3000 people, around 8000 people died within two weeks of gas release, injured more than 500,000 people. Similarly, recent Tsunamis spilled dangerous **radioactive materials** in surrounding areas of Fukushima, Japan. The accidents are compounded if they occur during transport/transit by bus/truck. Acute Exposure Guideline levels for selected Airborne Chemicals (AEGLs) are constantly revised and updated by Committee of Toxicology, USA. AGEL indicate threshold exposure limits for general public from ten minutes to eight hours. Depending upon the degree of toxicity and exposure period (10 min,30 min, 1 hr, 4 hr, 8 hr), three levels have been indicated - AGEL-1,AGEL-2,AGEL-3. The recently revised volume (20$^{th}$ volume) lists guidelines for n-propyl Chloroformate and isopropyl Chloroformate.

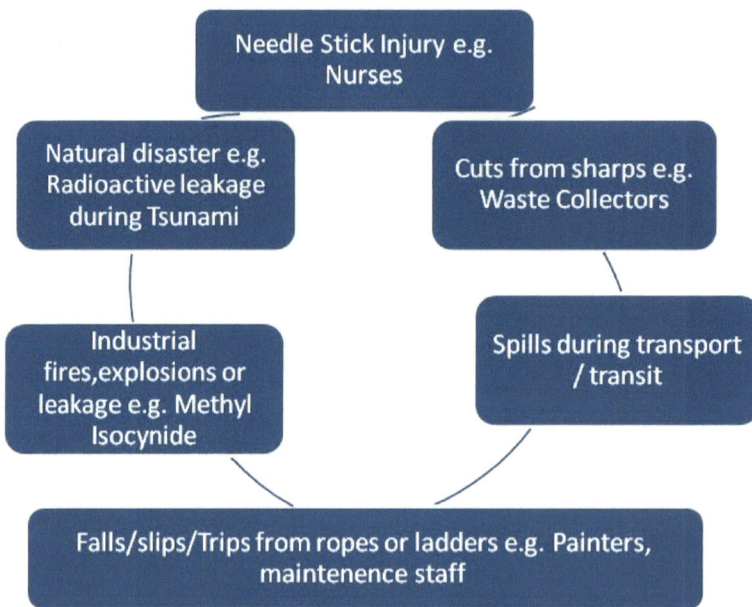

**Fig. (13).** Workplace disasters may lead to lifelong disability or death.

Worldwide, more than 2.5% HIV infections and 40% Hepatitis B and C infections amongst healthcare workers are due to needle stick injury. Reduction of **needle stick injury** is important, as re-injury is devastating. As the number of healthcare workers is small in developing countries like Tanzania and South Africa, such injuries lead to decrease in number of trained professionals. Therefore, information tools for reducing needle stick injury among healthcare workers is currently under test in countries like Vietnam in an NIH based project carried out by International Council of Nurses and WHO.

## Miscellaneous

### *The Effect of Various Occupations on Respiratory System*

High mortality has been widely reported in literature owing to respiratory failures (Fig. **14**) due to poor working conditions. The worker in industrial, non-industrial, agricultural setting or farm is exposed to dust, fumes or bio-aerosols. *Asthma* is a well-known occupational health hazard worldwide. Once a worker develops occupational asthma, recovery is difficult; symptoms continue years after the source of exposure is eliminated [70]. Occupational asthma is reported for sawmill workers, carpenters, *etc.* for Cedar wood, *Thujaplicata* [71]. Potroom asthma is recognised in Aluminium workers.

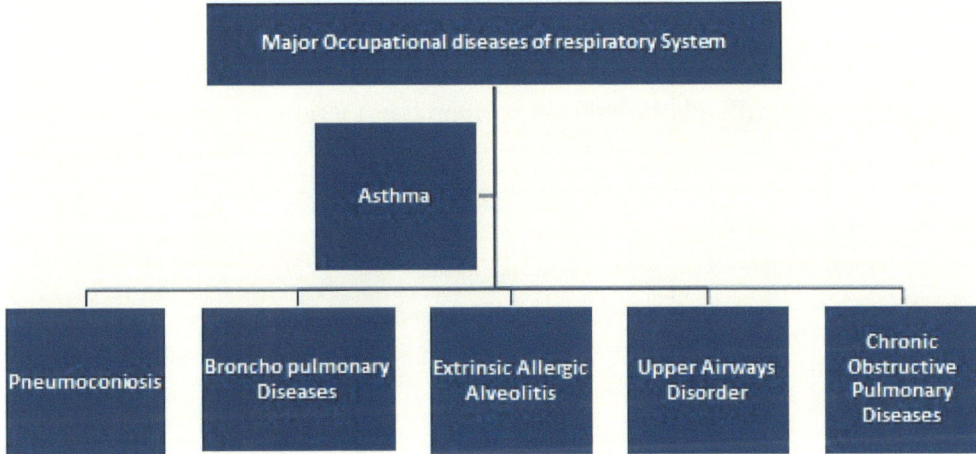

**Fig. (14).** Major occupational diseases of respiratory.

Asthma aggravated by work is also a recognised form of disease [72]. *Rhinitis* is an inflammatory disease of nasal passage. Work related and work exacerbated both types of Rhinitis are identified by panel of experts from European and non-European countries [72]. Several studies on united airways disease models show that occupational asthma and rhinitis are also interrelated especially when high molecular weight sensitizers are involved [73]. Despite high prevalence of Asthma, its wide socio-economic impact is underestimated. In order to diagnose Asthma serological testing is suggested.

The accumulation of dust in lungs generates a wide variety of respiratory disorders, particularly **pneumoconiosis.** There are various categories of dust (Figs **15** & **16**). **Organic dust** is dust from plant, animal or microbial origin. For example, dust generated during making of carpet or obtaining cotton from cotton plant would be considered dust of plant origin. **Inorganic dust** is dust obtained during extraction or processing or actual use of any mineral or metal. For example, dust generated during extraction/manufacture/use of Coal/cement/ aluminium. Besides microbially contaminated aerosols, there are various examples of dust, wood, textile and paper dust. While irritation of mucous membranes, chronic bronchitis, chronic obstructive pulmonary disease, rhinitis, inhalation fevers are other respiratory diseases associated with various professions [74]. There are a number of substances like plastics, resins, cement, batteries, dyes *etc.* which sensitise respiratory pathway. They are collectively termed as **Sa substances (Substances causing airway sensitisation)** [75]. Some substances act as both skin and airway sensitizers [70]. In several cases of occupational distress, extrinsic allergic alveolitis and lung damage occur due to irritating gases and smoke *e.g.* mists from contaminated oil lead to allergic alveolitis. Sometimes, chemical pneumonitis results from exposure to toxic fumes.

All the dust can be broadly classified into Inorganic or Organic Dust.

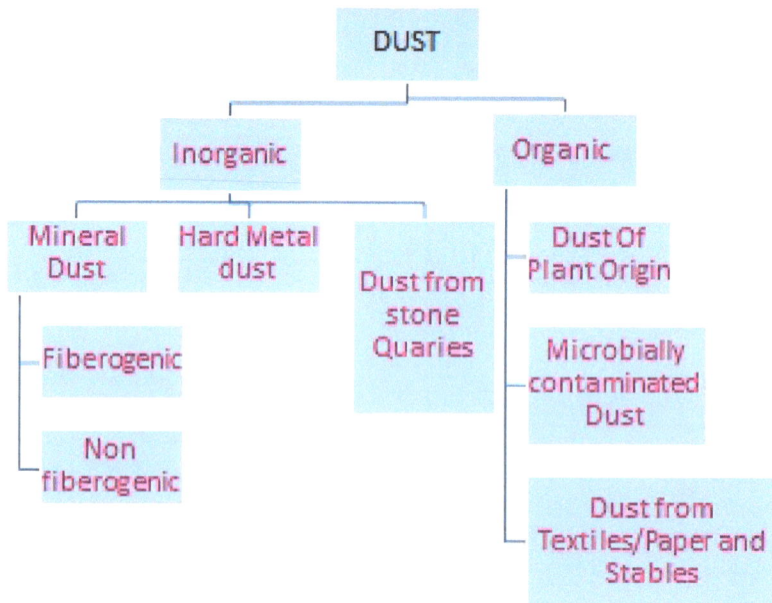

**Fig. (15).** Broad classification of types of dust.

## *Dusts of Inorganic Origin*

Inorganic dust is further divided into Mineral dust, hard metal dust and dust from quarries.

## *Mineral Dust*

There are two types of mineral dusts (Fig. **16**) *fibrogenic* mineral dust and *non-fibrogenic* mineral dust.

### *Fibrogenic Mineral Dust*

Strong fibrogenic mineral dusts are dusts from silica, asbestos, iron and coal. Fibrogenic dust causes *collagenous pneomoconioses* which is non-reversible and causes permanent harm to the structure of alveoli. *Silicosis* is caused by silica dust, *anthraco-silicosis* is caused by exposure to coal dust, *asbestosis* is caused by exposure to asbestos and *siderosis* is caused by exposure to iron dust. Silicosis is characterised by small nodules in lung parenchyma while asbestosis has characteristic irregular opaque areas at the base of lung [76].

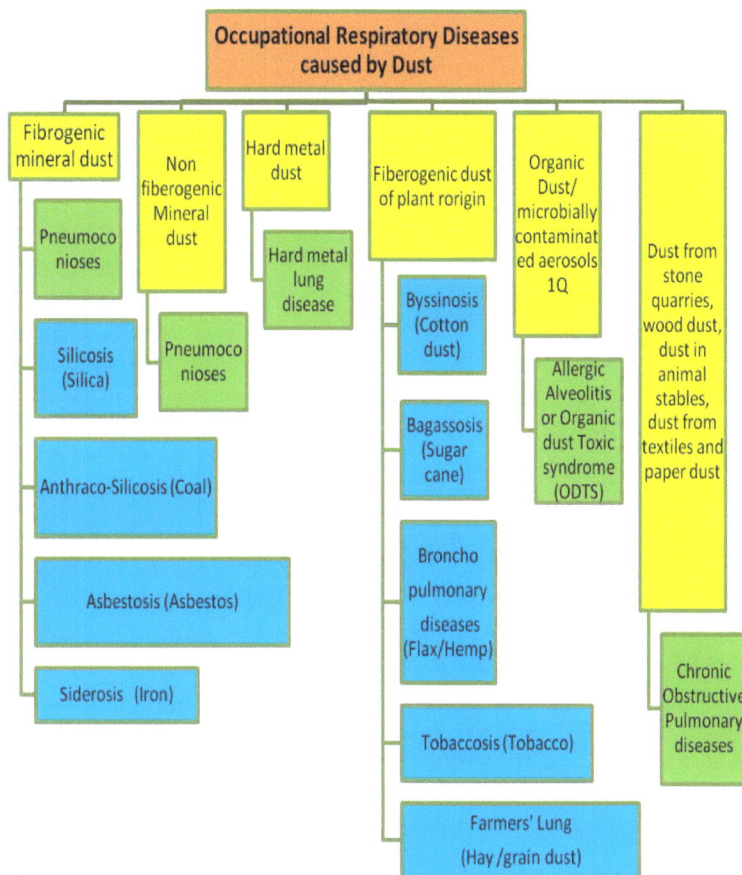

**Fig. (16).** Various types of respiratory diseases caused by dusts.

## Non-Fibrogenic Mineral Dust

This dust includes dust from talc, graphite, marble, gypsum, plaster of paris, cement *etc.* Non-fibrogenic dust causes *non-collagenous pneomoconioses* which is reversible and causes no harm to the structure of alveoli.

*Hard metal dust* comprises of fumes of Tungsten-carbide and cobalt or diamond-cobalt. The exposure to workers occurs when they process, manufacture or use tools composed of hard metal, Tungsten-carbide and cobalt or diamond-cobalt. It leads to hard metal lung disease characterised by multinucleated giant cells in alveoli leading to Giant Cell Interstitial Pneumonitis (GIP) [77].

## Dusts of Organic Origin

### Fibrogenic Dust of Plant Origin

Chronic loss of lung function is observed on long term inhalation of Cotton dust among cotton factory workers is called Byssinosis [78]. Lung dysfunction is observed on direct inhalation of sugar cane dust in sugarcane factory workers in India [79]. The alteration of lung function due to sugar cane dust is called Bagassosis.

*Inhalation Fevers*: They are mild diseases due to inhalation. Metal fume fever, polymer fume fever is all medically recognised flu like syndromes which develop on inhalation of metals like zinc oxide, oxides of copper, brass *etc.* and polymers like Polytetrafluoroethane commercially known as Teflon. Organic Dust Toxic Syndrome (ODTS)is another flu-like disease which occurs due to short term inhalation of any organic dust.

Workers involved in cement production, construction, stable, metallurgical smelting, textile, stone quarries, fertilizer, paper and pesticide industry are under risk of Chronic Obstructive Pulmonary Diseases (COPD). It is estimated that 10-20% cases of COPD are due to exposure to dust and irritant gases [80].

### Effects of Various Occupations on Skin

Skin is the first barrier to provide protection from physical, chemical or biological assaults. There are three types of skin diseases due to occupational exposure to various chemicals and environments (Fig. **17**). Skin diseases rank as the largest group of occupational diseases after musculoskeletal disorders. Occupational skin diseases have a tendency to become chronic as a twelve year follow up study in Sweden demonstrates [81]. The quality of patient life degrades and absentia from work enhances after minor skin problems turn chronic. The skin diseases can be mainly classified into three categories [82].

1. Direct Skin Effects
   These effects include irritation, necrosis and dermatitis.

2. Immune Mediated Skin Effects
   These include antibody mediated disorders like Urticaria or allergic contact dermatitis (ACD).

2. Systemic Effect
   This kind of effect manifest once the skin is sensitised and the burden of toxicity is high, other organs/system are affected *e.g.* Asthma, neurotoxicity, liver injury *etc.*

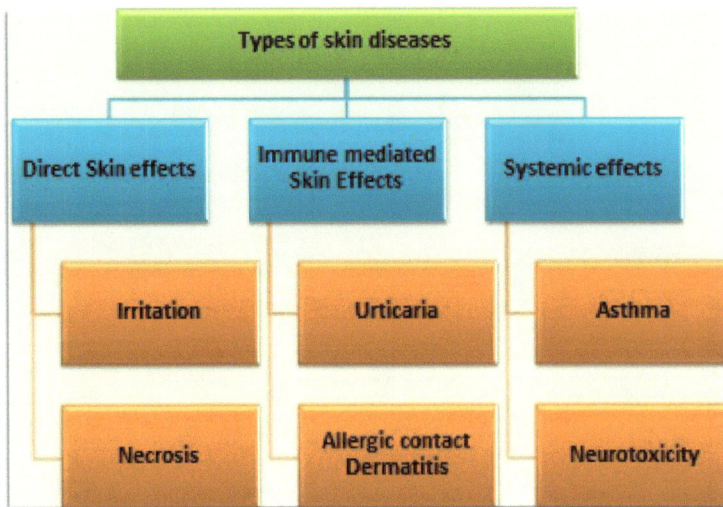

**Fig. (17).** Major occupational diseases of skin.

### *Wet Work*

It is defined as enhanced exposure to wet surface during work. For example, if a person immerses hand in liquid for more than two hours or washes hand for more than 20 times in a single working day, than the nature of his work would be considered as wet work. Constant wetting-drying cycles and frequent use of drying agents, detergents or antiseptics are a cause of hand skin diseases.

The 2010 International Labour Organization (ILO) list of occupational diseases lists following skin diseases (Figs **18** & **19**). Burn/frost bite and Acid/alkali corrosion/ulcer are additional skin diseases associated with work.

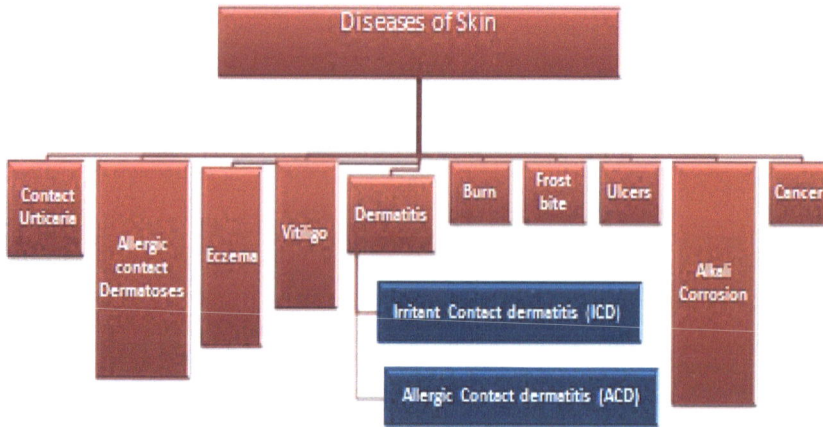

**Fig. (18).** Major occupational diseases of skin.

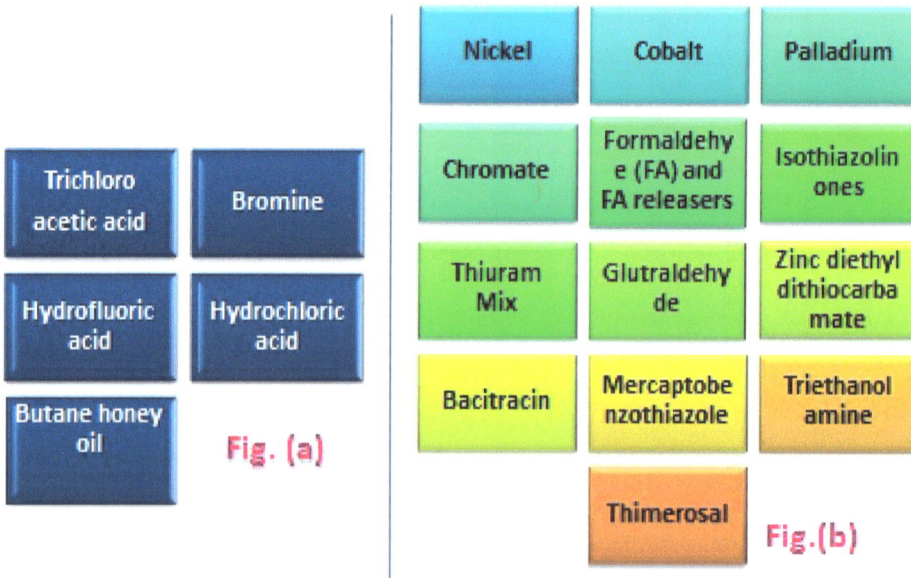

**Fig. (19).** Indicative list of chemical burns and allergic contact dermatitis causing substances.

## *Dermatitis*

The agents causing allergic contact dermatitis include metals, drugs, plant products, resins, wood allergens, plastic, rubber and glues [83], therefore all the workers dealing with these allergens are under potential threat of occupational disease. For instance, nursing and pharmacy staff is at occupational risk of contact dermatitis due to crushing of tablets particularly tetrazepam [84]. Besides, healthcare workers high risk occupations for Dermatitis include textile or leather industry workers, hair dressers and Construction workers. In a survey on occupational risk for dermatitis Carba mix, thiuram mix, epoxy resin, formaldehyde, and nickel were found to be most common allergens for both allergic and contact dermatitis [85]. Thiuram mix, carbamix, potassium dichromate and epoxy resin (Fig. **19-b**) are considered highest frequency allergens while blue collar work and wet work are other risk factors for development of *Irritant Contact dermatitis (ICD)* and *Allergic Contact dermatitis (ACD)* [86]. Activation of innate immune system by chemicals lead to Irritant Contact dermatitis (ICD) while delayed type hypersensitivity response leads to Allergic Contact dermatitis (ACD). Filaggrin gene codes for a protein which is involved in skin barrier function. Any mutation in Filaggrin gene makes a person more prone to development of occupational contact Dermatitis [87].

### *Contact Urticaria*

Frequent glove users like healthcare staff are under constant threat to Contact Urticaria due to latex allergy or due to physical pressure of the glove. This is commonly called as *Glove related hand Urticaria*. In Japan, Contact Urticaria is also caused by percutaneous sensitization to parvalbumin through physical contact with fish during work [88].

### *Vitiligo*

Selective destruction of melanocytes leads to depigmentation of skin, leading to disorder called Vitiligo. Vitiligo is developed in workers who are exposed to chemicals containing 4-hydroxy hydroquinone or alkyl phenol or catechol derivatives like agents for preventing emulsification of oil, deodorizing agents, copying papers, formaldehyde resins, phenolic disinfectants, rubber glue, automotive fuel additives, plasticizers for cellulose acetate, printing ink, lacquer, paint and resin [89].

### *Eczema*

Eczema is one of the most common skin diseases mostly associated with wet work. Occupational hand eczema is common for bakers, hair dressers, nursing staff particularly dental surgery assistants, cleaners, house hold workers, florist, metal workers, painters. A large number of apprentice nurses were found to develop eczema during training and had Filaggrin mutations [90, 91].

## *Allergic Contact Dermatitis*

It is an immune-mediated antigen-specific reaction of skin to chemicals like preservatives particularly present in cosmetics and industrial products. Nursing and health care staffs are more susceptible to Allergic Contact Dermatitis. Metals also act as allergen.

## *Cancer*

Occupational exposure to sun is a leading cause of skin cancers amongst farmers, engineers, construction workers *etc.* In some countries, educational programmes are designed to enhance awareness in workers, dermatologists *etc.* There are numerous substances at workplaces which cause cancer. They range from Heavy metals like arsenic, coal tars, wood dust, and radiations to aromatic compounds like Benzene (Fig. **20**). Study on offshore oil industry workers from Norway demonstrated that they are exposed to oil vapour from shaker, exhaust fumes, vapour from mixing chemicals used for drilling, natural gas. Chemicals used for processing make them a high risk population for cancer [92]. World health organization (WHO) constantly revises and adds new carcinogens to the list after strict evaluation. A detailed account of cancer causing agents is given in chapter **3**.

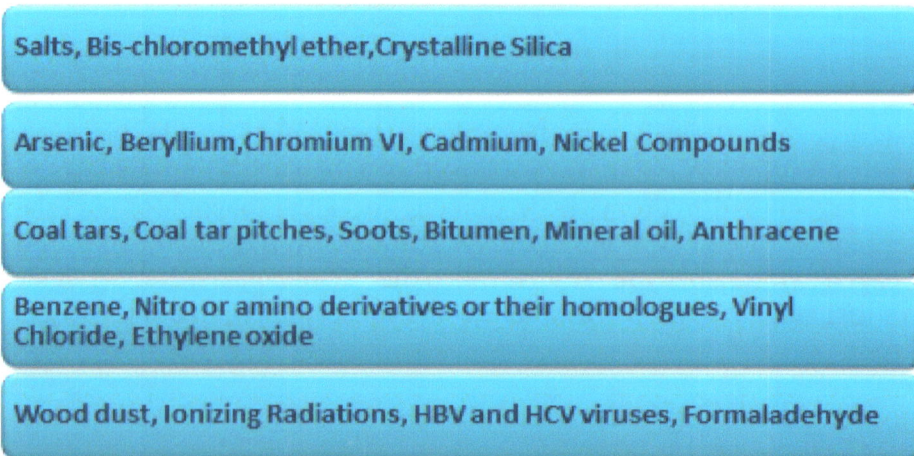

Salts, Bis-chloromethyl ether,Crystalline Silica

Arsenic, Beryllium,Chromium VI, Cadmium, Nickel Compounds

Coal tars, Coal tar pitches, Soots, Bitumen, Mineral oil, Anthracene

Benzene, Nitro or amino derivatives or their homologues, Vinyl Chloride, Ethylene oxide

Wood dust, Ionizing Radiations, HBV and HCV viruses, Formaladehyde

**Fig. (20).** Cancer causing agents at workplace.

## *Labor Laws and Organizations*

In 1911, **workman's compensation act** was established in Washington, **compensation law** was passed shortly thereafter, in the same year in Wisconsin.

It defined workers' right and safe employment practices for the first time to compensate for employees' wages. **WHO, ILO and members of European Union** (Fig. **21**) identify the Psychological health risks to workers. Netherlands Organization for applied Scientific Research (TNO) is the second largest Organization in Europe dedicated to applied research for improving quality of life, work and employment. Institute of Work, Health & Organizations(I-WHO) in U.K., Federal Institute of Occupational Safety and Health in Germany, National Institute for Occupational safety and Prevention in Italy [InstitutoSuperiore per la Prevenzione e La Sicurezza del Lavoro (ISPESL)] are other Organizations dedicated to study and research of occupational health. Central Institute for Labour Protection-National Research Institute, Poland [Centralny Instytut Ochrony Pracy-Panstwowy Instytut Badawczy (CIOP-PIB)] is the independent state Organization reviewing Occupational safety and solutions. Finnish Institute of Occupational Health (FIOH), Finland is one of the oldest European Organizations dedicated to study of working conditions at workplace. In United States, the Occupational Safety and Health Administration (OSHA) is responsible for establishing guidelines for workers. All these Organizations aim towards finding out issues related to workers' emotional, physical and economic well-being.

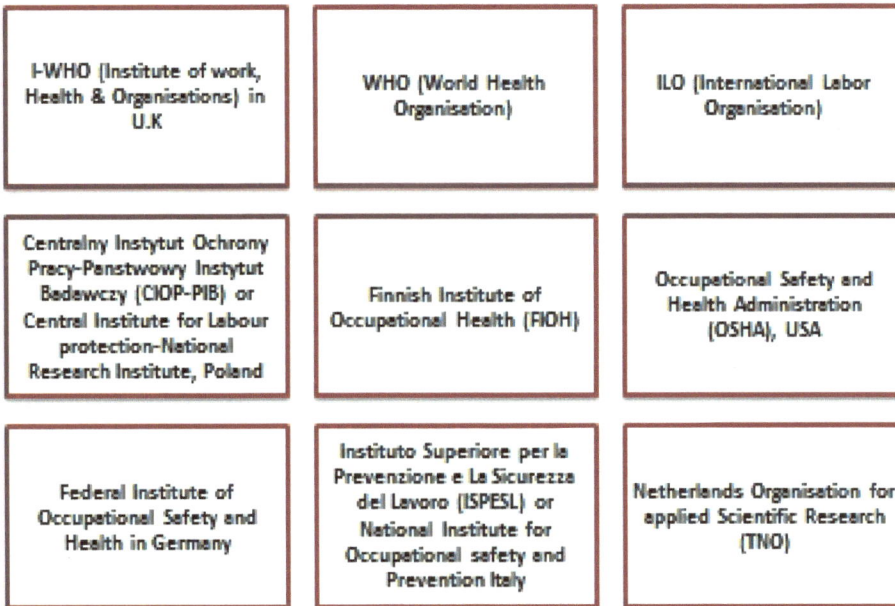

| I-WHO (Institute of work, Health & Organisations) in U.K | WHO (World Health Organisation) | ILO (International Labor Organisation) |
| --- | --- | --- |
| Centralny Instytut Ochrony Pracy-Panstwowy Instytut Badawczy (CIOP-PIB) or Central Institute for Labour protection-National Research Institute, Poland | Finnish Institute of Occupational Health (FIOH) | Occupational Safety and Health Administration (OSHA), USA |
| Federal Institute of Occupational Safety and Health in Germany | Instituto Superiore per la Prevenzione e La Sicurezza del Lavoro (ISPESL) or National Institute for Occupational safety and Prevention Italy | Netherlands Organisation for applied Scientific Research (TNO) |

**Fig. (21).** Premium organizations of the world dedicated to the cause of occupational health & safety.

## *World Health Organization(WHO)*

It is an organization of United Nations established in 1948.WHO'scharter was initially signed by 61 countries. Today, WHO has more than 160 country members and six regional offices. It tries to reach out to people through informative videos/talks/pictures on You tube, Facebook, Instagram and Twitter.

WHO is developing information tools, policies and guidelines to improve the critical difference between disability, illness, health and death of workers. It is working towards creating improved conditions by dispersing guidelines for unorganized sectors like agriculture or small scale industry or widely neglected high risk areas like mining [93].

WHO has adopted Occupational risk management tool box (Control Banding) developed by Health and safety Executive, England. It has an interactive software which provides information regarding safety procedures for managing workplace hazards. A tool kit for chemical exposures is developed and that can help prevent on-site injury with the help of the interactive software which provides solution according to the dose of a particular chemical, type and size of workplace. The software indicates about safer options for chemical use and safety requirements like ventilation, safety suits *etc.* according to the setting of work place. The solutions provided by the kit are affordable, easy to implement, being on-site, minimize risk of long term effect and follow up. Similar toolkits for Ergonomics, noise and psychosocial factors are also under consideration.

## *International Labour Organization (ILO)*

It was established in 1919.India was one of the founding members. Today, it has 186 strong members who meet in June every year. The members of the 106th International Labour Conference held on 5-16 June, 2017, Geneva, Switzerland deliberated on work issues related to conflict and war zones and Labour migration governance. The primary focus of **safe work** program by ILO is hazardous work like agriculture, construction, ship-breaking, mining which has either or all the three Ds - dirty, dangerous and difficult, particularly for children and young workers. The Organization has worked over the years and developed policy on radiation protection, popularly known as **recommendation 114**. The reports of ILO serve as resource for the rest of the world. For instance, 2014 outbreak of Ebola Virus in West-Africa was a public health emergency for healthcare workers as indicated by ILO.

## CONCLUSION

The current chapter tries to encompass the emerging disorders as the new occupations emerge creating previously unheard of maladies. The list of new age diseases and their causes is constantly revised every year by agencies like ILO and WHO as has been discussed previously in the chapter. The purpose of this chapter is to understand emerging diseases in order to work towards their prevention and cure. Sometimes, traditional measures of control need effective precautions in order to decrease the frequency.

## CONSENT FOR PUBLICATION

Not applicable.

## ACKNOWLEDGEMENTS

Declared none

## CONFLICT OF INTEREST

The author confirms that this chapter contents have no conflict of interest.

## REFERENCES

[1]     Douwes J, Thorne P, Pearce N, Heederik D. Bioaerosol health effects and exposure assessment: progress and prospects. Ann Occup Hyg 2003; 47(3): 187-200.
        [PMID: 12639832]

[2]     Alex A, Letizia M. Community-acquired methicillin-resistant Staphylococcus aureus: considerations for school nurses. J Sch Nurs 2007; 23(4): 210-3.
        [http://dx.doi.org/10.1177/10598405070230040501] [PMID: 17676968]

[3]     Newman KL, Newman LS. Occupational causes of sarcoidosis. Curr Opin Allergy Clin Immunol 2012; 12(2): 145-50.
        [http://dx.doi.org/10.1097/ACI.0b013e3283515173] [PMID: 22314258]

[4]     Ricci ML, Fontana S, Bella A, *et al.* Microbiologists of the Regional Agency for Environmental Protection of Novara. A preliminary assessment of the occupational risk of acquiring Legionnaires' disease for people working in telephone manholes, a new workplace environment for Legionella growth. Am J Infect Control 2010; 38(7): 540-5.
        [http://dx.doi.org/10.1016/j.ajic.2010.04.194] [PMID: 20472324]

[5]     Krogulska B, Matuszewska R, Bartosik M, Krogulski A, Szczotko M, Maziarka D. Respiratory symptoms among industrial workers exposed to water aerosol. A pilot study of process water and air microbial quality. Med Pr 2013; 64(1): 47-55.
        [PMID: 23650768]

[6]     Muzi G, Murgia N, Abbritti G, Tinozzi C, dell'Omo M. Respiratory diseases in confined non-industrial working environments. G Ital Med Lav Ergon 2006; 28(3): 276-8.
        [PMID: 17144417]

[7]     Mencke N. Future challenges for parasitology: vector control and 'One health' in Europe: the veterinary medicinal view on CVBDs such as tick borreliosis, rickettsiosis and canine leishmaniosis. Vet Parasitol 2013; 195(3-4): 256-71.
        [http://dx.doi.org/10.1016/j.vetpar.2013.04.007] [PMID: 23680539]

[8]     Mircean V, Dumitrache MO, Györke A, *et al.* Seroprevalence and geographic distribution of Dirofilaria immitis and tick-borne infections (Anaplasma phagocytophilum, Borrelia burgdorferi sensu

lato, and Ehrlichia canis) in dogs from Romania. Vector Borne Zoonotic Dis 2012; 12(7): 595-604.
[http://dx.doi.org/10.1089/vbz.2011.0915] [PMID: 22607068]

[9]     Chin TL, MacGowan AP, Jacobson SK, Donati M. Viral infections in pregnancy: advice for healthcare
        workers. J Hosp Infect 2014; 87(1): 11-24.
        [http://dx.doi.org/10.1016/j.jhin.2013.12.011] [PMID: 24767811]

[10]    Dutkiewicz J, Cisak E, Sroka J, Wójcik-Fatla A, Zając V. Biological agents as occupational hazards -
        selected issues. Ann Agric Environ Med 2011; 18(2): 286-93.
        [PMID: 22216801]

[11]    Lanier C, André V, Séguin V, *et al.* Recurrence of Stachybotrys chartarum during mycological and
        toxicological study of bioaerosols collected in a dairy cattle shed. Ann Agric Environ Med 2012;
        19(1): 61-7.
        [PMID: 22462447]

[12]    Hayes RB, van Nieuwenhuize JP, Raatgever JW, ten Kate FJ. Aflatoxin exposures in the industrial
        setting: an epidemiological study of mortality. Food Chem Toxicol 1984; 22(1): 39-43.
        [http://dx.doi.org/10.1016/0278-6915(84)90050-4] [PMID: 6537935]

[13]    Olsen JH, Dragsted L, Autrup H. Cancer risk and occupational exposure to aflatoxins in Denmark. Br
        J Cancer 1988; 58(3): 392-6.
        [http://dx.doi.org/10.1038/bjc.1988.226] [PMID: 3179193]

[14]    Foladi S, Hedayati MT, Shokohi T, Mayahi S. Study on fungi in archives of offices, with a particular
        focus on Stachybotrys chartarum. J Mycol Med 2013; 23(4): 242-6.
        [http://dx.doi.org/10.1016/j.mycmed.2013.09.003] [PMID: 24139181]

[15]    Reboux G, Piarroux R, Mauny F, *et al.* Role of molds in farmer's lung disease in Eastern France. Am J
        Respir Crit Care Med 2001; 163(7): 1534-9.
        [http://dx.doi.org/10.1164/ajrccm.163.7.2006077] [PMID: 11401869]

[16]    Biermaier B, Gottschalk C, Schwaiger K, Gareis M. Occurrence of Stachybotrys chartarum chemotype
        S in dried culinary herbs. Mycotoxin Res 2015; 31(1): 23-32.
        [http://dx.doi.org/10.1007/s12550-014-0213-3] [PMID: 25346283]

[17]    Viegas C, Faria T, Gomes AQ, Sabino R, Seco A, Viegas S. Fungal contamination in two Portuguese
        wastewater treatment plants. J Toxicol Environ Health A 2014; 77(1-3): 90-102.
        [http://dx.doi.org/10.1080/15287394.2014.866925] [PMID: 24555650]

[18]    Coggins MA, Hogan VJ, Kelly M, *et al.* Workplace exposure to bioaerosols in podiatry clinics. Ann
        Occup Hyg 2012; 56(6): 746-53.
        [PMID: 22291206]

[19]    Zielińska-Jankiewicz K, Kozajda A, Szadkowska-Stańczyk I. Occupational exposure to prions due to
        contact with meat and bone meal (MBM). Med Pr 2008; 59(1): 75-8.
        [PMID: 18663898]

[20]    Zahir F, Rizwi SJ, Haq SK, Khan RH. Low dose mercury toxicity and human health. Environ Toxicol
        Pharmacol 2005; 20(2): 351-60.
        [http://dx.doi.org/10.1016/j.etap.2005.03.007] [PMID: 21783611]

[21]    Rubens O, Logina I, Kravale I, Eglîte M, Donaghy M. Peripheral neuropathy in chronic occupational
        inorganic lead exposure: a clinical and electrophysiological study. J Neurol Neurosurg Psychiatry
        2001; 71(2): 200-4.
        [http://dx.doi.org/10.1136/jnnp.71.2.200] [PMID: 11459892]

[22]    Schwartz BS, Lee BK, Bandeen-Roche K, *et al.* Occupational lead exposure and longitudinal decline
        in neurobehavioral test scores. Epidemiology 2005; 16(1): 106-13.
        [http://dx.doi.org/10.1097/01.ede.0000147109.62324.51] [PMID: 15613953]

[23]    Catalani S, Rizzetti MC, Padovani A, Apostoli P. Neurotoxicity of cobalt. Hum Exp Toxicol 2012;
        31(5): 421-37.

[http://dx.doi.org/10.1177/0960327111414280] [PMID: 21729976]

[24]    Zhang Y, Zhang J. JiangX,Ni L, Ye C, Han C, Sharma K, Wang X. Hydroflouric acid (HF) in the western Zhejiang province of China: a 10 year epidemiological study. J Occup Med Toxicol 2016; 11: 55.
[http://dx.doi.org/10.1186/s12995-016-0144-3] [PMID: 27980604]

[25]    Green DR, Anthony TR. Occupational noise exposure of employees at locally-owned restaurants in a college town. J Occup Environ Hyg 2015; 12(7): 489-99.

[26]    Rabinowitz PM, Galusha D, Dixon-Ernst C, Clougherty JE, Neitzel RL. The dose-response relationship between in-ear occupational noise exposure and hearing loss. Occup Environ Med 2013; 70(10): 716-21.
[http://dx.doi.org/10.1136/oemed-2011-100455] [PMID: 23825197]

[27]    Basner M, Babisch W, Davis A, *et al.* Auditory and non-auditory effects of noise on health. Lancet 2014; 383(9925): 1325-32.
[http://dx.doi.org/10.1016/S0140-6736(13)61613-X] [PMID: 24183105]

[28]    Messingher G, Ryherd EE, Ackerman J. Hospital noise and staff performance. J Acoust Soc Am 2012; 132: 2031.
[http://dx.doi.org/10.1121/1.4755468]

[29]    Tomei G, Fioravanti M, Cerratti D, *et al.* Occupational exposure to noise and the cardiovascular system: a meta-analysis. Sci Total Environ 2010; 408(4): 681-9.
[http://dx.doi.org/10.1016/j.scitotenv.2009.10.071] [PMID: 19931119]

[30]    Yoon JH, Won JU, Lee W, Jung PK, Roh J. Occupational noise annoyance linked to depressive symptoms and suicidal ideation: a result from nationwide survey of Korea. PLoS One 2014; 9(8): e105321.
[http://dx.doi.org/10.1371/journal.pone.0105321] [PMID: 25144292]

[31]    Jovanović J, Jovanović M. The effect of noise and vibration on the cardiovascular system in exposed workers and possibilities of preventing their harmful effects. Med Pregl 1994; 47(9-10): 344-7.
[PMID: 7565325]

[32]    Turcot A, André Girard S, Courteau M, Baril J, Larocque R. Noise-induced hearing loss and combined noise and vibration exposure. Occup Med (Lond) 2015; 65(3): 238-44.
[http://dx.doi.org/10.1093/occmed/kqu214]

[33]    Futatsuka M, Sakurai T, Ariizumi M. Preliminary evaluation of dose-effect relationships for vibration induced white finger in Japan. Int Arch Occup Environ Health 1984; 54(3): 201-21.
[http://dx.doi.org/10.1007/BF00379050] [PMID: 6490180]

[34]    Bovenzi M, Zadini A, Franzinelli A, Borgogni F. Occupational musculoskeletal disorders in the neck and upper limbs of forestry workers exposed to hand-arm vibration. Ergonomics 1991; 34(5): 547-62.
[http://dx.doi.org/10.1080/00140139108967336] [PMID: 1653132]

[35]    Tucek M, Hlavkova J. Musculoskeletal disorders (MSDs) and working risk factors. Occup Environ Med 2014; A88(71) (Suppl. 1).
[http://dx.doi.org/10.1136/oemed-2014-102362.275]

[36]    Rosén B, Björkman A, Lundborg G. Improving hand sensibility in vibration induced neuropathy: A case-series. J Occup Med Toxicol 2011; 6(1): 13.
[http://dx.doi.org/10.1186/1745-6673-6-13] [PMID: 21524297]

[37]    Claudon M, Guillaume L. Diagnostic imaging and radiation hazards. Rev Prat 2015; 65(1): 79-81.
[PMID: 25842439]

[38]    Gérard JP. Occupational hazard related to ionizing radiation and surveillance of exposed peopleRev Prat. 2015; 65(1): 90-3.

[39]    Grajewski B, Whelan EA, Lawson CC, *et al.* Miscarriage among flight attendants. Epidemiology

2015; 26(2): 192-203.
[http://dx.doi.org/10.1097/EDE.0000000000000225] [PMID: 25563432]

[40]   Lim H, Agopian AJ, Whitehead LW, *et al.* National Birth Defects Prevention Study. Maternal occupational exposure to ionizing radiation and major structural birth defects. Birth Defects Res A Clin Mol Teratol 2015; 103(4): 243-54.
[http://dx.doi.org/10.1002/bdra.23340] [PMID: 25820072]

[41]   Walkosz BJ, Buller DB, Andersen PA, Wallis A, Buller MK, Scott MD. Factors Associated With Occupational Sun-Protection Policies in Local Government Organizations in Colorado. JAMA Dermatol 2015; 151(9): 991-7.
[http://dx.doi.org/10.1001/jamadermatol.2015.0575] [PMID: 25993051]

[42]   Xiang J, Bi P, Pisaniello D, Hansen A. Health impacts of workplace heat exposure: an epidemiological review. Ind Health 2014; 52(2): 91-101.
[http://dx.doi.org/10.2486/indhealth.2012-0145] [PMID: 24366537]

[43]   Kjellstrom T. Impact of climate conditions on occupational health and related economic Losses: A new feature of global and urban health in the context of climate change. Asia Pac J Public Health 2016; 28(2) (Suppl.): 28S-37S.
[http://dx.doi.org/10.1177/1010539514568711] [PMID: 25626424]

[44]   Horie S. Disorders caused by heat, cold, and abnormal pressure. Nihon Rinsho 2014; 72(2): 223-35.
[PMID: 24605519]

[45]   Xiang J, Bi P, Pisaniello D, Hansen A. The impact of heatwaves on workers' health and safety in Adelaide, South Australia. Environ Res 2014; 133: 90-5.
[http://dx.doi.org/10.1016/j.envres.2014.04.042] [PMID: 24906072]

[46]   Dehghan H, Mortazavi SB, Jafari MJ, Maracy MR. Cardiac strain comparison between workers with normal weight and overweight in the hot humid weather of the Persian Gulf region. J Educ Health Promot 2013; 2: 48.
[http://dx.doi.org/10.4103/2277-9531.119032] [PMID: 24251284]

[47]   McInnes A, Akram M, Macfarlane EM, Keeqel T, Sim MR, Smith P. Associations between high ambient temperature and acute work related case-crossover analysis using workers' compensation claims data. Scand J Work Environ Health 2016; 43(1): 86-94.
[http://dx.doi.org/10.5271/sjweh.3602]

[48]   Chen CJ, Dai YT, Sun YM, Lin YC, Juang YJ. Evaluation of auditory fatigue in combined noise, heat and workload exposure. Ind Health 2007; 45(4): 527-34.
[http://dx.doi.org/10.2486/indhealth.45.527] [PMID: 17878624]

[49]   Buzanello MR, Moro AR. Association between repetitive work and occupational cold exposure. Work 2012; 41(41) (Suppl. 1): 5791-3.
[PMID: 22317689]

[50]   Jammes Y, Delvolgo-Gori MJ, Badier M, Guillot C, Gazazian G, Parlenti L. One-year occupational exposure to a cold environment alters lung function. Arch Environ Health 2002; 57(4): 360-5.
[http://dx.doi.org/10.1080/00039890209601422] [PMID: 12530605]

[51]   Hassi J, Gardner L, Hendricks S, Bell J. Occupational injuries in the mining industry and their association with statewide cold ambient temperatures in the USA. Am J Ind Med 2000; 38(1): 49-58.
[http://dx.doi.org/10.1002/1097-0274(200007)38:1<49::AID-AJIM6>3.0.CO;2-3] [PMID: 10861766]

[52]   Thetkathuek A, Yingratanasuk T, Jaidee W, Ekburanawat W. Cold exposure and health effects among frozen food processing workers in eastern Thailand. Saf Health Work 2015; 6(1): 56-61.
[http://dx.doi.org/10.1016/j.shaw.2014.10.004] [PMID: 25830071]

[53]   Imray CH, Richards P, Greeves J, Castellani JW. Nonfreezing cold-induced injuries. J R Army Med Corps 2011; 157(1): 79-84.
[http://dx.doi.org/10.1136/jramc-157-01-14] [PMID: 21465916]

[54]  Mäkinen TM, Jokelainen J, Näyhä S, Laatikainen T, Jousilahti P, Hassi J. Occurrence of frostbite in the general population--work-related and individual factors. Scand J Work Environ Health 2009; 35(5): 384-93.
[http://dx.doi.org/10.5271/sjweh.1349] [PMID: 19730758]

[55]  Chaput B, Eburdery H, Courtade-Saïdi M, De Bonnecaze G, Grolleau JL, Garrido I. Freon gas frostbite: an unusual burn evolving in two stages. Chir Main 2012; 31(3): 166-9.
[http://dx.doi.org/10.1016/j.main.2012.04.004] [PMID: 22658586]

[56]  Cappaert TA, Stone JA, Castellani JW, Krause BA, Smith D, Stephens BA. National Athletic Trainers' Association. National Athletic Trainers' Association position statement: environmental cold injuries. J Athl Train 2008; 43(6): 640-58.
[http://dx.doi.org/10.4085/1062-6050-43.6.640] [PMID: 19030143]

[57]  Lee YI, Ye BJ. Underwater and hyperbaric medicine as a branch of occupational and environmental medicine. Ann Occup Environ Med 2013; 25(1): 39.
[http://dx.doi.org/10.1186/2052-4374-25-39] [PMID: 24472678]

[58]  Azizi MH. Ear disorders in scuba divers. Int J Occup Environ Med 2011; 2(1): 20-6.
[PMID: 23022815]

[59]  Guidotti TL. Occupational repetitive strain injury. Am Fam Physician 1992; 45(2): 585-92.
[PMID: 1739044]

[60]  Choobineh AR, Daneshmandi H, Aghabeigi M, Haghayegh A. Prevalence of musculoskeletal symptoms among employees of Iranian petrochemical industries: October 2009 to December 2012. Int J Occup Environ Med 2013; 4(4): 195-204.
[PMID: 24141868]

[61]  Belliveau MJ, Leung C, Abouammoh MA. Intravitreal injections inducing de quervain tenosynovitis: injector's wrist. Retin Cases Brief Rep 2015; 9(2): 149-50.
[http://dx.doi.org/10.1097/ICB.0000000000000121] [PMID: 25462130]

[62]  Giersiepen K, Spallek M. Carpal tunnel syndrome as an occupational disease. DtschArztebl Int 2011; 108(14): 238-428.

[63]  Blanc-Lapierre A, Rousseau MC, Weiss D, El-Zein M, Siemiatycki J, Parent MÉ. Lifetime report of perceived stress at work and cancer among men: A case-control study in Montreal, Canada. Prev Med 2017; 96: 28-35.
[http://dx.doi.org/10.1016/j.ypmed.2016.12.004] [PMID: 27923666]

[64]  Tjalvin G, Magerøy N, Bråtveit M, Lygre SH, Hollund BE, Moen BE. Odour as a determinant of persistent symptoms after a chemical explosion, a longitudinal study. Ind Health 2017; 55(2): 127-37.
[http://dx.doi.org/10.2486/indhealth.2016-0155] [PMID: 27916759]

[65]  Kumar M, Verma M, Das T, Pardeshi G, Kishore J, Padmanandan A. A study of workplace violence experienced by doctors and associated risk factors in a tertiary care hospital of South Delhi, India. J Clin Diagn Res 2016; 10(11): LC06-10.
[PMID: 28050406]

[66]  Yumang-Ross DJ, Burns C. Shift work and employee fatigue: implications for occupational health nursing. Workplace Health Saf 2014; 62(6): 256-61.
[PMID: 24971821]

[67]  Rothermund E, Kilian R, Rottler E, *et al.* Improving Access to Mental Health Care by Delivering Psychotherapeutic Care in the Workplace: A Cross-Sectional Exploratory Trial. PLoS One 2017; 12(1): e0169559.
[http://dx.doi.org/10.1371/journal.pone.0169559] [PMID: 28056101]

[68]  Berriault CJ, Lightfoot NE, Seilkop SK. Conard BRInjury mortality in a cohort of mining, smelting, and refining workers in Ontario. Arch Environ Occup Health 2016; 30: 1-11.

[69]    Jeong BY, Lee S, Lee JD. Workplace accidents and work-related illnesses of household waste collectors. Saf Health Work 2016; 7(2): 138-42.
[http://dx.doi.org/10.1016/j.shaw.2015.11.008] [PMID: 27340601]

[70]    Montano D. Chemical and biological work-related risks across occupations in Europe: a review. J Occup Med Toxicol 2014; 9: 28.
[http://dx.doi.org/10.1186/1745-6673-9-28] [PMID: 25071862]

[71]    Jacobsen G, Schaumburg I, Sigsgaard T, Schlunssen V. Non-malignant respiratory diseases and occupational exposure to wood dust. Part I. Fresh wood and mixed wood industry. Ann Agric Environ Med 2010; 17(1): 15-28.
[PMID: 20684477]

[72]    Moscato G, Vandenplas O, Van Wijk RG, *et al.* European Academy of Allergology and Clinical Immunolgy.EAACI position paper on occupational rhinitis. Respir Med 2009; 103(2): 201-8.
[PMID: 18980836]

[73]    Ameille J, Hamelin K, Andujar P, *et al.* Occupational asthma and occupational rhinitis: the united airways disease model revisited. Occup Environ Med 2013; 70(7): 471-5.
[http://dx.doi.org/10.1136/oemed-2012-101048] [PMID: 23390199]

[74]    Latza U, Baur X. Occupational obstructive airway diseases in Germany: Frequency and causes in an international comparison. Am J Ind Med 2005; 48(2): 144-52.
[http://dx.doi.org/10.1002/ajim.20186] [PMID: 16032736]

[75]    Schnuch A, Lessmann H, Schulz KH, *et al.* When should a substance be designated as sensitizing for the skin ('Sh') or for the airways ('Sa')? Hum Exp Toxicol 2002; 21(8): 439-44.
[http://dx.doi.org/10.1191/0960327102ht278oa] [PMID: 12412637]

[76]    McLoud TC. Occupational lung disease. Radiol Clin North Am 1991; 29(5): 931-41.
[PMID: 1871262]

[77]    Nemery B, Verbeken EK, Demedts M. Giant cell interstitial pneumonia (hard metal lung disease, cobalt lung). Semin Respir Crit Care Med 2001; 22(4): 435-48.
[http://dx.doi.org/10.1055/s-2001-17386] [PMID: 16088691]

[78]    Christiani DC, Wang XR. Respiratory effects of long-term exposure to cotton dust. Curr Opin Pulm Med 2003; 9(2): 151-5.
[http://dx.doi.org/10.1097/00063198-200303000-00010] [PMID: 12574696]

[79]    Patil SN, Somade PM, Joshi AG. Pulmonary function tests in sugar factory workers of Western Maharashtra (India). J Basic Clin Physiol Pharmacol 2008; 19(2): 159-66.
[http://dx.doi.org/10.1515/JBCPP.2008.19.2.159] [PMID: 19024932]

[80]    Wiszniewska M, Lipińska-Ojrzanowska A, Ziemba K, Walusiak-Skorupa J. Chronic obstructive pulmonary disease--work-related disease. Med Pr 2012; 63(2): 217-28.
[PMID: 22779328]

[81]    Meding B, Lantto R, Lindahl G, Wrangsjö K, Bengtsson B. Occupational skin disease in Sweden--a 12-year follow-up. Contact Dermat 2005; 53(6): 308-13.
[http://dx.doi.org/10.1111/j.0105-1873.2005.00731.x] [PMID: 16364116]

[82]    Anderson SE, Meade BJ. Potential health effects associated with dermal exposure to occupational chemicals. Environ Health Insights 2014; 8 (Suppl. 1): 51-62.
[PMID: 25574139]

[83]    Swinnen I, Goossens A. An update on airborne contact dermatitis: 2007-2011. Contact Dermat 2013; 68(4): 232-8.
[http://dx.doi.org/10.1111/cod.12022] [PMID: 23343440]

[84]    Swinnen I, Ghys K, Kerre S, Constandt L, Goossens A. Occupational airborne contact dermatitis from benzodiazepines and other drugs. Contact Dermat 2014; 70(4): 227-32.

[http://dx.doi.org/10.1111/cod.12166] [PMID: 24289767]

[85]    Rietschel RL, Mathias CG, Fowler JF Jr, *et al.* North American Contact Dermatitis Group. Relationship of occupation to contact dermatitis: evaluation in patients tested from 1998 to 2000. Am J Contact Dermat 2002; 13(4): 170-6.
[http://dx.doi.org/10.1053/ajcd.2002.36635] [PMID: 12478531]

[86]    Coman G, Zinsmeister C, Norris P. Occupational Contact Dermatitis: Workers' Compensation Patch Test Results of Portland, Oregon, 2005-2014. Dermatitis 2015; 26(6): 276-83.
[http://dx.doi.org/10.1097/DER.0000000000000142] [PMID: 26551607]

[87]    Kasemsarn P, Bosco J, Nixon RL. The Role of the Skin Barrier in Occupational Skin Diseases. Curr Probl Dermatol 2016; 49: 135-43.
[http://dx.doi.org/10.1159/000441589] [PMID: 26844905]

[88]    Sano A, Yagami A, Suzuki K, *et al.* Two cases of occupational contact urticaria caused by percutaneous sensitization to parvalbumin. Case Rep Dermatol 2015; 7(2): 227-32.
[http://dx.doi.org/10.1159/000439080] [PMID: 26464568]

[89]    Ahn YS, Kim MG. Occupational skin diseases in Korea. J Korean Med Sci 2010; 25 (Suppl.): S46-52.
[http://dx.doi.org/10.3346/jkms.2010.25.S.S46] [PMID: 21258591]

[90]    Visser MJ, Verberk MM, van Dijk FJ, Bakker JG, Bos JD, Kezic S. Wet work and hand eczema in apprentice nurses; part I of a prospective cohort study. Contact Dermat 2014; 70(1): 44-55.
[http://dx.doi.org/10.1111/cod.12131] [PMID: 24102246]

[91]    Visser MJ, Verberk MM, Campbell LE, *et al.* Filaggrin loss-of-function mutations and atopic dermatitis as risk factors for hand eczema in apprentice nurses: part II of a prospective cohort study. Contact Dermat 2014; 70(3): 139-50.
[http://dx.doi.org/10.1111/cod.12139] [PMID: 24102300]

[92]    Stenehjem JS, Friesen MC, Eggen T, Kjærheim K, Bråtveit M, Grimsrud TK. Self-reported Occupational Exposures Relevant for Cancer among 28,000 Offshore Oil Industry Workers Employed between 1965 and 1999. J Occup Environ Hyg 2015; 12(7): 458-68.
[http://dx.doi.org/10.1080/15459624.2014.989358] [PMID: 25671393]

[93]    wwwwhoint/occupational_health/publications/newsletter/en/

CHAPTER 2

# Occupational Hazards as Neurological Disorders

**Rajesh Singh Yadav**[1] and **Kumar Vaibhav**[2,*]

[1] *Department of Criminology and Forensic Science, School of Applied Sciences, Dr. Harisingh Gour Central University, Sagar 470 003 (MP), India*

[2] *Department of Neurosurgery, Augusta University, 1120 15th St, Augusta 30912 (GA), USA*

**Abstract:** Human brain is the most complex organ that controls various complicated functions like behavior, learning, talking, memorizing, organizing, listening, performance of routine skills and interaction with environment. The vulnerability of brain towards toxic effects of occupational hazards is very high due to the presence of high amount of polyunsaturated fatty acids and high metabolism. Interference with xenobiotics or occupational hazards disrupts homeostatic processes and may cause long lasting effects in humans including behavioural abnormalities, cognitive deficits, depression and movement disorders. Prolonged exposure to toxicants and occupational hazards leads to altered membrane and lipid rafts leading to various neurological disorders including Parkinson's and Alzheimer's disease. Therefore, a deep knowledge of occupation induced hazards mediated alteration on normal brain development and function will add to the research of minimizing this risk. In the present chapter, different occupational hazards are discussed with their deleterious effects on human brain.

**Keywords:** Brain, Occupational hazards, Pesticides, Heavy metals, Industrial chemicals, Radiation, Neurological disorders, Stress, Oxidative stress, Toxicity, Alzheimer's disease, Parkinson's disease, Neurobehavior.

## INTRODUCTION

Human brain is the most complex organ involved in various complicated functions and controls behavior, learning, talking, memorizing, organizing, listening, performance of routine skills and interaction with environment [1]. Development of brain in human occurs both during the prenatal and early postnatal periods through the process of synchronized and concurrent milestones that do not occur during any other life stages. This developmental process occurs through the proliferation and migration of cells and transformed into correct cell type via the process of neurogenesis, differentiation and synaptogenesis. At the

* **Corresponding author Kumar Vaibhav:** Department of Neurosurgery, Augusta University, 1120 15th St, Augusta 30912 (GA), USA; Tel: +1 706 721 6331; Fax: +1 706 721 8293; Email: kvaibhav@augusta.edu

**Farhana Zahir (Ed.)**

same time the organogenesis and refined neural circuits are also formed through the process of apoptosis [2]. The different neurotransmitter systems in brain are developed at different time point and associated with the various functions including pharmacological and physiological activities in our body. Alteration or disruption in any of these processes or steps following exposure to toxic chemicals including neurotoxicants may cause long lasting effects in humans including neurobehavioural abnormalities, cognitive deficits, depression and movement disorders [1, 3 - 6]. In addition, interference by xenobiotics or occupational hazards during this period may also cause malformation of the brain [7, 8]. The developing nervous system was found to be more susceptible to neurotoxic insults of pesticides than adult animals due to toxico-kinetic differences, small body size, different ratio of fat, muscle and water, higher breathing and metabolic rate and immature enzymatic machinery (Fig. **1**) [3, 9, 10]. Besides, immature blood brain barrier also facilitates the neurotoxic chemicals to cross the placental barrier from mother to fetus which is an important factor of early life exposure in developing individuals and responsible for neurological disorders [11, 12].

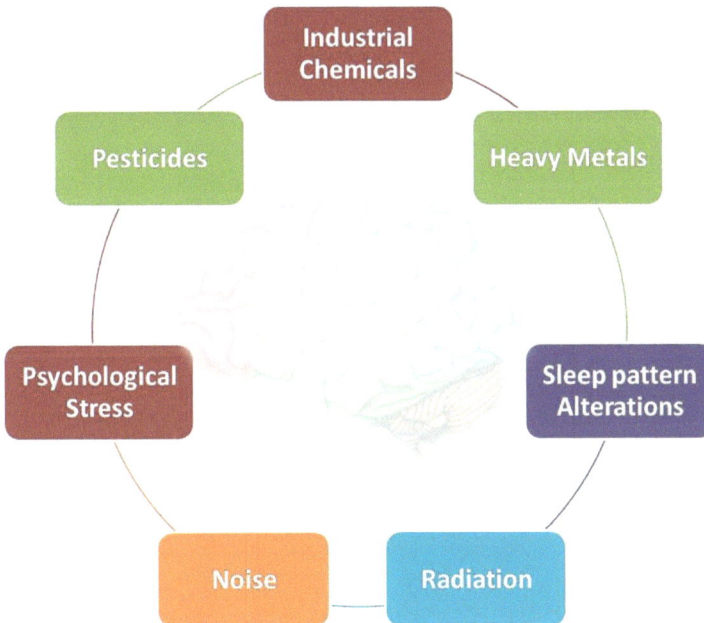

**Fig. (1).** Schematic representation of various factors present at occupational and non-occupational settings which may contribute to neurological and neuropsychiatric disorders.

The vulnerability of brain towards toxic effects of occupational hazards is very high due to the presence of high amount of polyunsaturated fatty acids that are the easy targets of the reactive oxygen species. These reactive species damage the lipid membrane and alter the composition of lipid rafts leading to various neurological disorders including Parkinson's and Alzheimer's disease [13]. There are a million of children working in hazardous situations all over the world and are at serious risk due to pesticides and other neurotoxic chemicals (Fig. **2**). It has been estimated that only in South Asia about 44 million children are involved in child labor [14].

| | |
|---|---|
| **Lead** | • Industrial waste materials, used in building construction, lead-acid batteries, bullets and shot, weights, pewters, fusible alloys and as a radiation shield |
| **Arsenic** | • Contaminated ground water, copper smelter workers, gallium arsenite, computer chips, pesticides manufacturing |
| **Mercury** | • CFLs, dental filling, Gold workers, contaminated fishes, industrial waste materials. |
| **Thallium** | • Electronics industry, pharmaceutical industry, glass manufacturing, infrared detectors and also in nuclear medicine scan |
| **Manganese** | • Treatment for rust and corrosion prevention on steel, in industries as pigments, as oxidizers, as the cathode material in zinc-carbon and alkaline batteries |
| **Carbon disulfide** | • Spinning process to make artificial silk thread from pulp, building block in organic chemistry, as an industrial and chemical non-polar solvent |
| **Phthalates** | •Plasticizers, coatings of pharmaceutical tablets, stabilizers, dispersants, lubricants and suspending agents. Other applications include adhesives and glues, electronics, agricultural adjuvants, building materials, medical devices, children's toys, printing inks and coatings, food products and textiles. |
| **Polychlorinated biphenyl** | • Dielectric and coolant fluids, electrical apparatus, cutting fluids for machining operations, carbon paper and in heat transfer fluids |
| **Pesticides** | • Through uses in homes, gardens, agriculture to protect crops and public health programmes |
| **Radiations** | • Industrial radiography, medical radiology and nuclear medicine, uranium mining, nuclear power plant and research laboratories |

**Fig. (2).** Occupational and Non-occupational sources of various heavy metals, industrial chemicals, pesticides and radiation associated with the neurodevelopmental and neurological disorders.

## OCCUPATIONAL HAZARDS

An occupational exposure could be defined as the exposure occurs during the performance of duties at the industries, agriculture and other places which may place a worker at risk of infection and associated health effects. There are convincing evidences suggested that the chemicals present in the environment could be a potential source of occupational exposure to humans which may interrupt neurodevelopmental processes during the critical windows (Fig. **2**). Epidemiological studies related to occupational exposure are mainly associated with the adverse neurotoxic effects of occupational hazards including metals (lead, mercury, arsenic and cadmium), polychlorinated biphenyls, pesticides, solvents and other industrial chemicals and radiation on humans [13, 15 - 17]. In the recent years, job stress at work place mainly business process outsourcing (BPO) call centers has been found to be a great cause of occupational hazards leading to depression, anxiety and neuropsychiatric disturbances in the individuals. [18]

## Pesticides

Pesticides considered as the major occupational hazards and pollution causing agents. Their Indiscriminate and excessive use become a matter of concern through the world [19 - 21]. The production of pesticides and their uses pattern in homes, gardens and agriculture to protect crops and public health programs have been increased tremendously in recent years [21 - 23]. India is the second largest manufacturer of pesticides in Asia after China and ranked twelfth globally [23, 24]. On the basis of pesticides' use, they are categorized as insecticides, fungicides, herbicides and rodenticides and based on their mechanisms of action they are broadly classified as organophosphates, pyrethroids, carbamates and organochlorines [20]. A new class of insecticides known as neonicotinoids which are chemically related to nicotine has been recently introduced and their use has grown significantly in the past decade. According to a study published in Science magazine, neonicotinoids are affecting bee colonies near farmland by reducing their survival percentage, but also impair its natural social defense system [25]. Human could be exposed to pesticides through occupational uses during manufacturing, application on crops, harvesting, handling of crops and public health programs [26, 27]. Further, the presence of high levels of pesticide residues in food products including vegetables, cereals and fruits enhances the risk of exposure of general population and associated adverse outcomes (Fig. **3**) [28, 29]. The cases of mental retardation, neurobehavioral and developmental have also been reported in offspring where selected exposures of pesticides occur during pregnancy even in low amount [29 - 31]. Adverse consequences including neurotoxic alterations in the workers exposed through occupational medicine has also been reported [27]. In all the Asian countries agriculture still remains an important sector. Hence, for the production of quality food the use of pesticides is also increased,  leading to occupational health hazards. Studies have revealed that exposure to pesticides damages the brain circuitry and alter the behavioral and neurological functions in exposed individuals [29 - 33]. Long term exposure of pesticides caused memory deficits, disorientation, irritability, confusion, speech difficulties, insomnia and extra-pyramidal symptoms [28, 34]. Individuals exposed to pesticides demonstrated that the long-term exposure may leads to the development of vascular diseases, decrease in the activity of butyrylcholinesterase and acetylcholinesterase, alterations in haematological parameters associated with the enhanced oxidative stress [23, 35, 36].

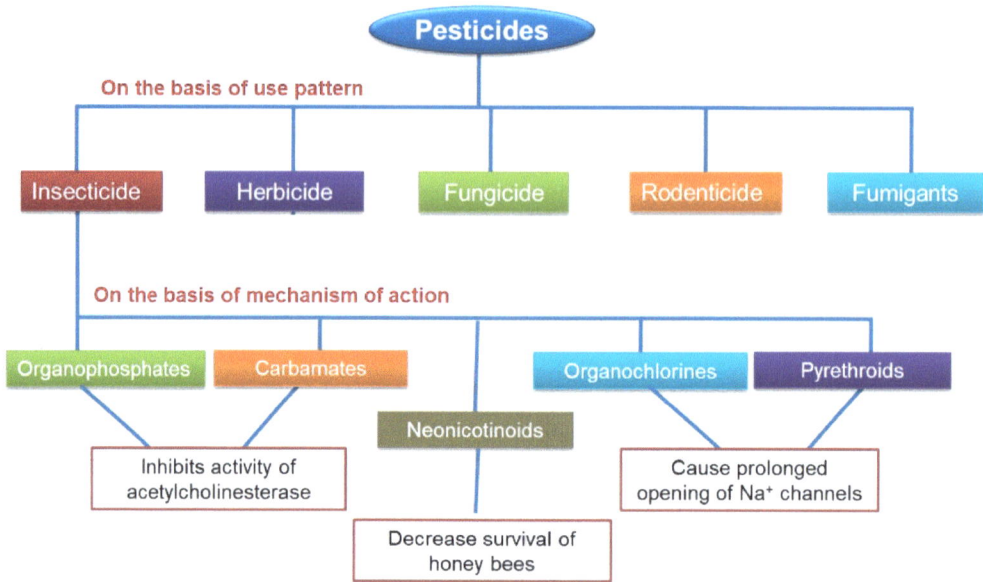

**Fig. (3).** Classification of Pesticides on the bases of their use pattern and mechanism of action. Organophosphates and carbamates showed their toxic effects by inhibiting the enzyme acetylcholinesterase while organochlorines and pyrethroids affects the opening of sodium channels. New class of insecticides, called as neonicotinoids decreases survivals of honey bees by diminishing their social defense. But it's effect on humans is still unknown.

Risk factor in the etiology of various neurodegenerative diseases including Parkinson's disease, dementia and Alzheimer's disease have been found to be enhanced following exposure to pesticides including organophosphates and pyrethroids in occupational workers [37 - 40]. Studies on biological monitoring by estimating levels of pesticides and their metabolites in exposed individuals have also been carried out to understand their burden and associated risk [41]. Impaired neurobehavioral and neuropsychological functions have been reported in pesticide exposed individuals [29, 32, 33], especially, children and infants are found to be more vulnerable [3, 42]. Due to the high production and using pattern of organophosphates, human exposure is quite imminent and linked with various neurological disorders. Incidences of human exposure to organophosphates are therefore frequent both under occupational and non-occupational conditions due to their indiscriminate and excessive use [43 - 46]. High residues of organophosphate compounds including monocrotophos has been detected in the blood of individuals and children residing in villages and associated neurobehavioral abnormalities have aroused a great concern among the health scientists [26, 47 - 49]. Enhanced oxidative stress as a measure of lipid peroxidation following exposure to monocrotophos in rats and its association with cholinergic and dopaminergic deficits has also been reported [50, 51]. Lein *et al.*, suggested that there should be translational research to understand the detailed mechanism of neurobehavioral toxicity with repeated occupational exposures to organophosphates [52]. They also suggested the research strategy for identifications of biomarkers in organophosphates neurotoxicity.

Due to the high bio-efficacy and easy biodegradable ability, pyrethroids are now widely used in agriculture, in homes and gardens and in veterinary practices to control ectoparasites [53]. Their use has been potentially increased as compared to organophosphorus insecticides due to their wide safety margins [53 - 55]. Alone in vector control program the use of active ingredients of synthetic pyrethroids has been estimated over 520 tons annually in all over the world [56]. Based on their structure pyrethroids are classified into two types known as type I and type II [57, 58]. Due to their structural dissimilarities, type I pyrethroids produce T syndrome linked with ataxia, tremors, hyperexcitation, convulsions while type II pyrethroids produce CS syndrome associated with choreoathetosis, salivation, hyperactivity and paralysis [59]. Multiple mechanisms have been suggested in the neurotoxicity of pyrethroids which affects various sites in central nervous system and cause neurobehavioural and neurochemical alterations [60 - 62]. These pyrethroids alters sodium and chloride channels and depolarize the membrane and cause apoptosis in nerve cells associated with other cellular effects including hyperexcitability and conduction block [63]. There effects have also been reported on mitochondrial membrane potentials leading to increase oxidative stress and cellular damage. The symptoms including dizziness, headache, consciousness, convulsive attacks, nausea, anorexia, fatigue, increased stomal secretion and pulmonary edema have been reported following exposure to pyrethroids [64]. Exposure to lambda-cyhalothrin, a type II synthetic pyrethroid in rats has been found to cause learning and memory deficits and motor disorder associated with the enhanced oxidative stress [61, 62]. Besides organophosphates and pyrethroids, several other groups of pesticides including carbamates and organochlorines are also used by the human hence, enhance their risk of exposure and associated health effects. Children have been found to have higher exposure than adolescent and adults due to their immature BBB and inefficient metabolic activity [5, 65] as evident by the presence of pyrethroids metabolites in the urine of pregnant women which further establish a link with adverse pregnancy outcomes [66 - 68]. As a result of occupational exposure, metabolites of pyrethroids have also been found in the urine of school children [69].

## Industrial Chemicals and Heavy Metals

Due to industrialization, the neurotoxic diseases through occupational exposure have become incremental in recent years. The pattern of these disorders has been changed from organophosphate to heavy metal intoxication and also from organic solvent to semiconductor agent poisoning. Liu *et al.*, in a review suggested the correlation of neurological diseases with the timeline of industrial development in Taiwan [70]. They reported that neurological manifestations may be transient or permanent and may range from cognitive dysfunction, cerebellar ataxia, Parkinsonism, sensorimotor neuropathy and autonomic dysfunction to neuromuscular junction disorders. In their review they studied the occupational neurotoxins from 1968 to 2012 in which 16 occupational neurotoxins, including organophosphates, toxic gases, heavy metals, organic solvents and other toxic chemicals were included. Epidemiological evidence suggested that exposure to solvents, metals, asphyxiates and other substances in humans are associated with an increased risk of ototoxicity either in presence or absence of noise exposure [70].

Lead, methylmercury, arsenic, thallium, manganese are the potential heavy metals, and polychlorinated biphenyls (PCBs), n-hexane, toluene, tetramethyl ammonium hydroxide and dimethylamine borane are industrial chemicals that have been studied in association with the neurotoxic effects in prenatally exposed children and adults. Studies have been reported that low level exposures to lead, methyl- mercury, arsenic and PCBs may impair the neurobehavioral development including cognition in children [71, 72]. Julvez and Graandjean reviewed and performed epidemiological studies on female workers and neurodevelopment of their children and reported the vulnerability of the developing brain to occupational hazards like lead and methylmercury which could be associated with neurobehavioral impairments in the progeny [1]. Studies have reported that the development of the chemical industry leads to the contribution of new chemical compounds including phthalates, BPA, TBBPA, and PCBs into the environment. These chemicals easily reached to the living cells, accumulate in the tissues and body organs and cause health problems. These chemical compounds were also found to affect the neurogenesis and synaptic transmission process linked with neurodegenerative diseases due to their ability to cross placental barrier and the blood-brain barrier [73]. Woimant and Trocello [74] in their studies discussed the role of heavy metals in the physiology and pathology of the nervous system and suggested that their deficiency or accumulation may lead to severe neurodegeneration. Caserta *et al.* [75], studied the effect of heavy metals including lead, mercury and cadmium on infant health including neurological, developmental and endocrine disorders. They reported the presence of heavy metals in placental tissues, amniotic fluid and umbilical cord blood which might have caused bad impact on fetuses and later children's health. Lead, a heavy metal is a known neurotoxicant involved in the etiology of Alzheimer's disease, Parkinson's disease, schizophrenia, brain damage, mental retardation and many behavioral problems. Exposure to lead has been found to be associated with the damage in the prefrontal cerebral cortex, hippocampus and cerebellum linked with various neurological disorders [76].

Arsenic compounds are used in the manufacture of insecticides, fungicides, herbicides and antifouling paints [77, 78]. These are also used in the pharmaceutical and glass industries and in the manufacture of sheep-dips, leather preservatives and poisonous baits which can be a potential source of occupational exposure to human [79 - 81]. Gallium arsenide and indium arsenide are used in the production of certain semiconductor devices such as field-effect transistors and microwave integrated circuits and in optoelectronics. High levels of arsenic in ground water in certain regions of Asian countries (India, China, Bangladesh, Nepal, Taiwan, Myanmar and Thailand) and many other regions of the globe (South America, Mexico, Argentina and Chile) are cause of concern due to associated health problems in humans [82 - 84]. High levels of arsenic have been reported in carbonate spring waters in New Zealand, Romania and the United States (0.4–1.3 mg/l), artesian wells in Taiwan and China (up to 1.8 mg/l) and groundwater in Cordoba, Argentina (up to 3.4 mg/l) and India (up to 3.2 mg/l). Exposure of general population to arsenic has also been reported through folk medicines and by consuming contaminated sea food [85 - 87]. Further, consumption of arsenic contaminated food is quite common in regions having high levels of arsenic in ground water and thus, serves as a potential source of arsenic exposure [88 - 91].

Occupational exposure to arsenic occurs primarily among workers involved in copper smelting [92], burning arsenic-rich coal in power plants [93] and using pesticides containing arsenic [94]. The soil can be heavily contaminated (more than 90 mg/kg) with arsenic in close vicinity of copper smelting units [95]. The median concentration of arsenic in soil and dust has been found 502 and 857 mg/kg near smelting unit in San Luis Potosi, Mexico. The median concentration of arsenic in the urine of children living nearby was 196 µg/g of creatinine (range 69–594 µg/g of creatinine). Exposure to arsenic through inhalation may also occur during production of gallium arsenide in the microelectronics industry, demolition of oil-fired boilers and metal ore mining [96, 97]. Epidemiological studies have revealed that chronic arsenic exposure to humans affects both the central and peripheral nervous system including peripheral neuropathy [82, 87, 98]. Alterations in motor behavior, impaired learning and concentration, neurological and cognitive deficits are the common CNS manifestations reported following arsenic exposure in humans [99 - 104]. Gharibzadeh and Hoseini suggested that arsenic exposure might be a risk factor for Alzheimer's disease by inducing apoptosis in cortical neurons [105]. Children residing near the areas contaminated with arsenic and lead have been found to have impaired cognitive development. Further, it was found that arsenic exposure combined with lead may have synergistic effect [101]. Long term exposure to arsenic was associated with neurobehavioral dysfunctions in adolescents [106]. Studies also revealed that exposure to arsenic may cause serious implications such as social instability, social discrimination and family related problems in humans [82, 84, 107].

Kim suggested that carbon disulfide could be another source of occupational exposure [108]. Peoples involved in the spinning process to make artificial silk thread from pulp dissolved in a carbon disulfide solution were diagnosed with carbon disulfide poisoning. A study carried out on the ex-employees of that company reported that among 117 cases of chronic carbon disulfide poisoning there were 61.5% of workers with neurological and 15.4% with psychiatric disorders [109]. Lim *et al.*, first time reported the manganese poisoning through welding rods manufacturer crushing ferromanganese [110]. A number of cases of manganese induced Parkinsonism has been reported in welder workers after this incident [111]. Some of the industrial chemical such as lead, styrene, toluene and trichloroethylene has been found to cause ototoxicity in clinical and pre-clinical studies. Further, carbon monoxide and toluene appear to aggravate noise-induced hearing dysfunction [112]. Recently, Guthrie *et al.*, in their preliminary epidemiological studies have suggested that jet propulsion fuel-8, a kerosene-based fuel may interact with noise to induce hearing loss [113]. Further in experimental studies, they found that it damaged to presynaptic sensory cells in the cochlea which did not directly affected the peripheral auditory function but was associated with the brainstem dysfunction. On the other hand, food items derived from unfermented soybean products has been found to be associated with the deleterious effect in many individuals including incidences of Alzheimer's disease and dementia [114].

## Radiation Exposure

The occupational exposure of radiation to human and its associated adverse health effects are an alarming situation for the health scientists. The sources of occupational radiation exposure include the industrial radiography, medical radiology and nuclear medicine, uranium mining, nuclear power plant and research laboratories [115, 116]. The human beings could also be exposed to radiation from consumer products like tobacco (polonium-210), building materials, combustible fuels (gas, coal, *etc.*), ophthalmic glass, televisions, airport X-ray systems, smoke detectors, electron tubes and lantern mantles (thorium). The high levels of radiation exposure to human can cause visually dramatic radiation burns and also death through acute radiation syndrome. The effects of ionizing radiation on human health are generally dose dependent and hence considered as deterministic. The adverse health effects include cancer, teratogenesis, cognitive impairments and cardiovascular disease. The high levels of occupational exposure may result into radiation burns, acute and chronic radiation syndrome and radiation-induced thyroiditis. Exposure to mobile radiation in rats was found to cause detrimental effects as evident by decrease relative brain weight, neuronal damage, altered antioxidant status in brain and initiation of apoptotic cell death [117].

Several studies have reported that radiation may cause adverse effects on brain activity and behavior, gene expression and DNA, cell growth, proliferation and tumors, hormones, proteins and enzymes [118 - 123]. The other effects include decreased testosterone levels in men, miscarriages in pregnant women, birth defects in babies, Alzheimer's disease, cataracts, depression and suicides [124]. Kesari *et al.*, demonstrated that the deleterious health effects following exposure to radiation have been associated with increased ROS which may enhance the effect of microwave radiations and cause brain tumors, genotoxic effects, immune system deregulation, allergic and inflammatory responses, infertility, cardiovascular effects and neurodegenerative disorders [17]. They further suggested that the regular and long-term use of microwave devices (mobile phone, microwave oven) at domestic level can have negative impact upon biological system especially on brain [17]. The abnormal somatic effects such as cancer may be induced through exposure of radiation which may be manifested after years [116 - 124]. In addition, radiation exposure during developmental period showed teratogenic effects that could be observed as congenital malformation. For example, mobile phone induced electromagnetic radiation acted as a contributory factor in the development of oxidative stress in brain and liver injury in growing rats [125]. Similarly, total-body exposure to 0, 1, 2 and 3 Gray (Gy) (60) Co γ-rays significantly increased the expression of inflammatory genes such as Il1f10, Il17, Tnfrsf11b, Tnfsf12, Il12b and Il1f8 in mice brain. Further, the expression of pro-apoptotic gene Bik and nitric oxide synthase were also increased in radiation exposed mice, suggesting its adverse effects on molecular level [126].

## Stress and Neurological Disorders

Stress has long been linked with the cause of neuropsychiatric and neurological disorders. Hazards from occupational stress have long been a concern for the MNCs, call centers, companies and also health care industry. This occupational stress has been found to cause psychological distress in the individuals and it is reflected in the form of burnout, malingering, employee intent to leave, reduced patient satisfaction and diagnosis and treatment errors. The stress itself causes health problems but at the same time it also plays an important role in the contribution of neurotoxicity of various pesticides and industrial chemicals. It has been shown that the permeability of blood brain barrier increases during the stress condition and hence, increases the susceptibility of exposure towards various neurotoxins [127]. Studies have been reported that health care workers have higher rates of substance abuse and suicide than other professions and hence increased rates of depression and anxiety associated with job stress [128]. According to National Institute for Occupational Safety and Health (NIOSH), occupational stress is the harmful physical and emotional response that occur when the requirements of the job do not match the capabilities, resources, or needs of the worker [129]. It has been shown that a low amount of stress is beneficial as it alerts the minds to accomplish the complicated tasks but at the same time too much stress may severely affect the functioning of our brain and cause psychiatric and neurological disorders. Alterations in sleep patterns have been considered as the first symptom of too much stress which could be later associated with the neurological health problems including altered behavioral, rapid mood swings, lashing out or volatile temper, nervousness, anxiety, inability to concentrate and excessive worry. The other common symptoms of stress include headaches, restlessness, loss of appetite, dizziness and sexual impotence.

Studies have reported that stress is a contributory factor for the releasing of hormones and their impact on neuronal development. Recently, stress induced alterations in growth factors like neurotrophins, in particular brain-derived neurotrophic factor (BDNF), have been significantly involved in the modulation of stress induced pathology [129]. Long working hours associated with cardiovascular disease, obesity, hypertension, diabetes and shortening of sleep hours could be a linked with the life style related health problems which might be further coupled with neuroendocrine activation and associated neurological disorders [130]. In another study, Koyama reported a significant correlation of stress with the insomnia, depression, fatigue, chronic pain which may sometimes lead to suicide tendencies in individuals [131]. They further suggested the method of early detection of depression based on an interview regarding the sleep of workers which could be used in occupational health practice [131]. Alongwith the various health effects of stress, the altered neurogenesis is considered as the potential modulator in stress induced such effects [132]. Stress induced depression has also been found to be associated with the decreased neurogenesis [133]. Besides neurological symptoms, work stress has increased risk for cardiovascular diseases [130, 134]. In addition, occupational exposure through drug / medication has been associated with the neurotoxicity and adverse neurological symptoms. Psychosis is the most common issue in cases of drug abuse and have an adverse reaction during withdrawal of the drug [135].

## PREVENTION AND CONTROL

The risk of human exposure to pesticides and other industrial chemicals is enhanced several times in developing countries as safety regulations are less stringent and hazards of these toxins are not well understood. There is a need to develop the protective measures for workers occupationally exposed to toxic chemicals, ionizing radiation and job stress. To avoid the increasing risk towards these contributing factors and associated incidence of adverse biological effects, regulatory agencies should impose occupational exposure limits on adults and minors. To reduce the risk from radioactive substances they should be confined in the smallest possible space and kept out of the environment. There are several ways to cope with stress including exercise and yoga. On the other hand, the use of stimulants such as caffeine, nicotine and some narcotics should be avoided which may result the slow production of corticosteroids. Help from professional psychiatrists can assist in altering the way to deal with the adverse effects of stress. Further, invasive research on molecular basis may improve the understanding of mechanism of toxicity from occupational hazards and hence will be useful to develop protective measures. The awareness program about industrial hygiene could promote occupational safety and health care during the process of industrialization which may help developing countries from the risk of occupational hazards. Besides, employee assistance program may also be useful for health promotion and fitness to aware the peoples towards physical and mental well beings that affected through occupational exposure and decelerate their work efficiency. However, it is truly said 'Prevention is better than Cure'. By limiting the stress at work place, by minimizing the pollutants/toxicants exposure and by avoiding hazards, the incidences of neurological disorders can be reduced to minimum.

## CONSENT FOR PUBLICATION

Not applicable.

## ACKNOWLEDGEMENTS

Declared none.

## CONFLICT OF INTEREST

The author confirms that this chapter contents have no conflict of interest.

## REFERENCES

[1]     Julvez J, Grandjean P. Neurodevelopmental toxicity risks due to occupational exposure to industrial chemicals during pregnancy. Ind Health 2009; 47(5): 459-68.
[http://dx.doi.org/10.2486/indhealth.47.459] [PMID: 19834254]

[2]     Bartkowska K, Turlejski K, Grabiec M, Ghazaryan A, Yavruoyan E, Djavadian RL. Adult neurogenesis in the hedgehog (Erinaceus concolor) and mole (Talpa europaea). Brain Behav Evol 2010; 76(2): 128-43.
[http://dx.doi.org/10.1159/000320944] [PMID: 21079393]

[3]     Miodovnik A. Environmental neurotoxicants and developing brain. Mt Sinai J Med 2011; 78(1): 58-77.
[http://dx.doi.org/10.1002/msj.20237] [PMID: 21259263]

[4]     Rice D, Barone S Jr. Critical periods of vulnerability for the developing nervous system: evidence from humans and animal models. Environ Health Perspect 2000; 108 (Suppl. 3): 511-33.
[PMID: 10852851]

[5]     Sinha C, Seth K, Islam F, *et al.* Behavioral and neurochemical effects induced by pyrethroid-based mosquito repellent exposure in rat offsprings during prenatal and early postnatal period. Neurotoxicol Teratol 2006; 28(4): 472-81.
[http://dx.doi.org/10.1016/j.ntt.2006.03.005] [PMID: 16842967]

[6]     Grandjean P, Landrigan PJ. Neurobehavioural effects of developmental toxicity. Lancet Neurol 2014; 13(3): 330-8.
[http://dx.doi.org/10.1016/S1474-4422(13)70278-3] [PMID: 24556010]

[7]     Rogers JM, Kavlock RL. Developmental toxicology. Casaret and Doull's Toxicology: the Basic Science of Poisons. New York: McGraw-Hill 1996; pp. 301-31.

[8]     Dorman DC, Allen SL, Byczkowski JZ, *et al.* Methods to identify and characterize developmental neurotoxicity for human health risk assessment. III: pharmacokinetic and pharmacodynamic considerations. Environ Health Perspect 2001; 109 (Suppl. 1): 101-11.
[PMID: 11250810]

[9]     Renwick AG. Toxicokinetics in infants and children in relation to the ADI and TDI. Food Addit Contam 1998; 15 (Suppl.): 17-35.
[http://dx.doi.org/10.1080/02652039809374612] [PMID: 9602909]

[10]    Ginsberg G, Hattis D, Sonawane B, *et al.* Evaluation of child/adult pharmacokinetic differences from a database derived from the therapeutic drug literature. Toxicol Sci 2002; 66(2): 185-200.
[http://dx.doi.org/10.1093/toxsci/66.2.185] [PMID: 11896285]

[11]    Akhtar N, Srivastava MK, Raizada RB. Transplacental disposition and teratogenic effects of chlorpyrifos in rats. J Toxicol Sci 2006; 31(5): 521-7.
[http://dx.doi.org/10.2131/jts.31.521] [PMID: 17202764]

[12]    Eskenazi B, Rosas LG, Marks AR, *et al.* Pesticide toxicity and the developing brain. Basic Clin Pharmacol Toxicol 2008; 102(2): 228-36.
[http://dx.doi.org/10.1111/j.1742-7843.2007.00171.x] [PMID: 18226078]

[13]    Yadav RS, Tiwari NK. Lipid integration in neurodegeneration: an overview of Alzheimer's disease. Mol Neurobiol 2014; 50(1): 168-76.
[http://dx.doi.org/10.1007/s12035-014-8661-5] [PMID: 24590317]

[14]    UNICEF. Child labour 2015 Aug 27; Available from: http://www.unicef.org/protection/index_childlabour.html

[15]    Winneke G. Developmental aspects of environmental neurotoxicology: lessons from lead and polychlorinated biphenyls. J Neurol Sci 2011; 308(1-2): 9-15.
[http://dx.doi.org/10.1016/j.jns.2011.05.020] [PMID: 21679971]

[16]    Jurewicz J, Polańska K, Hanke W. Chemical exposure early in life and the neurodevelopment of children an overview of current epidemiological evidence. Ann Agric Environ Med 2013; 20(3): 465-86.
[PMID: 24069851]

[17]    Kesari KK, Siddiqui MH, Meena R, Verma HN, Kumar S. Cell phone radiation exposure on brain and associated biological systems. Indian J Exp Biol 2013; 51(3): 187-200.
[PMID: 23678539]

[18]    Padma V, Anand NN, Gurukul SMGS, Javid SMASM, Prasad A, Arun S. Health problems and stress in Information Technology and Business Process Outsourcing employees. J Pharm Bioallied Sci 2015; 7 (Suppl. 1): S9-S13.
[http://dx.doi.org/10.4103/0975-7406.155764] [PMID: 26015763]

[19]    Abdollahi M, Ranjbar A, Shadnia S, Nikfar S, Rezaie A. Pesticides and oxidative stress: a review. Med Sci Monit 2004; 10(6): RA141-7.
[PMID: 15173684]

[20]    Kumar A, Sharma B, Pandey RS. Toxicological assessment of pyrethroid insecticides with special reference to cypermethrin and lambda-cyhalothrin in freshwater fishes. Int J Biol Med Res 2010; 1: 315-25.

[21]    Joshi AK, Rajini PS. Hyperglycemic and stressogenic effects of monocrotophos in rats: evidence for the involvement of acetylcholinesterase inhibition. Exp Toxicol Pathol 2012; 64(1-2): 115-20.
[http://dx.doi.org/10.1016/j.etp.2010.07.003] [PMID: 20674316]

[22]    Abhilash PC, Singh N. Pesticide use and application: an Indian scenario. J Hazard Mater 2009; 165(1-3): 1-12.
[http://dx.doi.org/10.1016/j.jhazmat.2008.10.061] [PMID: 19081675]

[23]    Wafa T, Nadia K, Amel N, *et al.* Oxidative stress, hematological and biochemical alterations in farmers exposed to pesticides. J Environ Sci Health B 2013; 48(12): 1058-69.
[http://dx.doi.org/10.1080/03601234.2013.824285] [PMID: 24007483]

[24]    Aktar MW, Sengupta D, Chowdhury A. Impact of pesticides use in agriculture: their benefits and hazards. Interdiscip Toxicol 2009; 2(1): 1-12.
[http://dx.doi.org/10.2478/v10102-009-0001-7] [PMID: 21217838]

[25]    Tsvetkov N, Samson-Robert O, Sood K, *et al.* Chronic exposure to neonicotinoids reduces honey bee health near corn crops. Science 2017; 356(6345): 1395-7.
[http://dx.doi.org/10.1126/science.aam7470] [PMID: 28663503]

[26]    Costa LG, Giordano G, Guizzetti M, Vitalone A. Neurotoxicity of pesticides: a brief review. Front Biosci 2008; 13: 1240-9.
[http://dx.doi.org/10.2741/2758] [PMID: 17981626]

[27]    Dewan A, Rajendran TP. Asia WHOROfS-E Health implications from monocrotophos use: a review of the evidence in India: World Health Organization. Regional Office for South-East Asia 2009.

[28]    Melnyk LJ, Byron MZ, Brown GG, Clayton CA, Michael LC. Pesticides on household surfaces may influence dietary intake of children. Environ Sci Technol 2011; 45(10): 4594-601.
[http://dx.doi.org/10.1021/es104190k] [PMID: 21517066]

[29]    Harari R, Julvez J, Murata K, *et al.* Neurobehavioral deficits and increased blood pressure in school-age children prenatally exposed to pesticides. Environ Health Perspect 2010; 118(6): 890-6.
[http://dx.doi.org/10.1289/ehp.0901582] [PMID: 20185383]

[30]    Engel SM, Wetmur J, Chen J, *et al.* Prenatal exposure to organophosphates, paraoxonase 1, and cognitive development in childhood. Environ Health Perspect 2011; 119(8): 1182-8.
[http://dx.doi.org/10.1289/ehp.1003183] [PMID: 21507778]

[31]    Bouchard MF, Chevrier J, Harley KG, *et al.* Prenatal exposure to organophosphate pesticides and IQ in 7-year-old children. Environ Health Perspect 2011; 119(8): 1189-95.
[http://dx.doi.org/10.1289/ehp.1003185] [PMID: 21507776]

[32]    Roldán-Tapia L, Parrón T, Sánchez-Santed F. Neuropsychological effects of long-term exposure to organophosphate pesticides. Neurotoxicol Teratol 2005; 27(2): 259-66.

[http://dx.doi.org/10.1016/j.ntt.2004.12.002] [PMID: 15734277]

[33]   Mackenzie Ross SJ, Brewin CR, Curran HV, Furlong CE, Abraham-Smith KM, Harrison V. Neuropsychological and psychiatric functioning in sheep farmers exposed to low levels of organophosphate pesticides. Neurotoxicol Teratol 2010; 32(4): 452-9.
[http://dx.doi.org/10.1016/j.ntt.2010.03.004] [PMID: 20227490]

[34]   Salvi RM, Lara DR, Ghisolfi ES, Portela LV, Dias RD, Souza DO. Neuropsychiatric evaluation in subjects chronically exposed to organophosphate pesticides. Toxicol Sci 2003; 72(2): 267-71.
[http://dx.doi.org/10.1093/toxsci/kfg034] [PMID: 12660361]

[35]   Arnal N, Astiz M, de Alaniz MJT, Marra CA. Clinical parameters and biomarkers of oxidative stress in agricultural workers who applied copper-based pesticides. Ecotoxicol Environ Saf 2011; 74(6): 1779-86.
[http://dx.doi.org/10.1016/j.ecoenv.2011.05.018] [PMID: 21700338]

[36]   Astiz M, Arnal N, de Alaniz MJT, Marra CA. Occupational exposure characterization in professional sprayers: clinical utility of oxidative stress biomarkers. Environ Toxicol Pharmacol 2011; 32(2): 249-58.
[http://dx.doi.org/10.1016/j.etap.2011.05.010] [PMID: 21843806]

[37]   Hancock DB, Martin ER, Mayhew GM, *et al.* Pesticide exposure and risk of Parkinson's disease: a family-based case-control study. BMC Neurol 2008; 8: 6.
[http://dx.doi.org/10.1186/1471-2377-8-6] [PMID: 18373838]

[38]   Wingo TS, Rosen A, Cutler DJ, Lah JJ, Levey AI. Paraoxonase-1 polymorphisms in Alzheimer's disease, Parkinson's disease, and AD-PD spectrum diseases. Neurobiol Aging 2012; 33(1): 204.e13-5.
[http://dx.doi.org/10.1016/j.neurobiolaging.2010.08.010] [PMID: 20947215]

[39]   Wang A, Costello S, Cockburn M, Zhang X, Bronstein J, Ritz B. Parkinson's disease risk from ambient exposure to pesticides. Eur J Epidemiol 2011; 26(7): 547-55.
[http://dx.doi.org/10.1007/s10654-011-9574-5] [PMID: 21505849]

[40]   Das K, Ghosh M, Nag C, *et al.* Role of familial, environmental and occupational factors in the development of Parkinson's disease. Neurodegener Dis 2011; 8(5): 345-51.
[http://dx.doi.org/10.1159/000323797] [PMID: 21346317]

[41]   Terry AV Jr, Gearhart DA, Beck WD Jr, *et al.* Chronic, intermittent exposure to chlorpyrifos in rats: protracted effects on axonal transport, neurotrophin receptors, cholinergic markers, and information processing. J Pharmacol Exp Ther 2007; 322(3): 1117-28.
[http://dx.doi.org/10.1124/jpet.107.125625] [PMID: 17548533]

[42]   Schroeder S. Mental retardation and developmental disabilities influenced by environmental neurotoxic insults. Environ Health prospect 2000; 108: 395-99.

[43]   Simcox NJ, Camp J, Kalman D, *et al.* Farmworker exposure to organophosphorus pesticide residues during apple thinning in central Washington State. Am Ind Hyg Assoc J 1999; 60(6): 752-61.
[http://dx.doi.org/10.1080/00028899908984498] [PMID: 10635541]

[44]   McCauley SR, Levin HS, Vanier M, *et al.* The neurobehavioural rating scale-revised: sensitivity and validity in closed head injury assessment. J Neurol Neurosurg Psychiatry 2001; 71(5): 643-51.
[http://dx.doi.org/10.1136/jnnp.71.5.643] [PMID: 11606677]

[45]   Curl CL, Fenske RA, Kissel JC, *et al.* Evaluation of take-home organophosphorus pesticide exposure among agricultural workers and their children. Environ Health Perspect 2002; 110(12): A787-92.
[http://dx.doi.org/10.1289/ehp.021100787] [PMID: 12460819]

[46]   Fenske RA, Hidy A, Morris SL, Harrington MJ, Keifer MC. Health and safety hazards in Northwest agriculture: setting an occupational research agenda. Am J Ind Med 2002; 2 (Suppl. 2): 62-7.
[http://dx.doi.org/10.1002/ajim.10081] [PMID: 12210684]

[47]   Mathur HB, Agarwal HC, Johnson S, Saikia N. Analysis of Pesticide residues in blood samples from villages of Punjab. CSE Report 2005. CSE/PML/PR-21/2005. Available from

http://www.cseindia.org/userfiles/Punjab_blood_report.pdf

[48]    Bjørling-Poulsen M, Andersen HR, Grandjean P. Potential developmental neurotoxicity of pesticides used in Europe. Environ Health 2008; 7: 50.
[http://dx.doi.org/10.1186/1476-069X-7-50] [PMID: 18945337]

[49]    Srivastava S, Narvi SS, Prasad SC. Levels of select organophosphates in human colostrum and mature milk samples in rural region of Faizabad district, Uttar Pradesh, India. Hum Exp Toxicol 2011; 30(10): 1458-63.
[http://dx.doi.org/10.1177/0960327110396525] [PMID: 21247996]

[50]    Sankhwar ML, Yadav RS, Shukla RK, *et al.* Impaired cholinergic mechanisms following exposure to monocrotophos in young rats. Hum Exp Toxicol 2012; 31(6): 606-16.
[http://dx.doi.org/10.1177/0960327111405860] [PMID: 21508071]

[51]    Sankhwar ML, Yadav RS, Shukla RK, *et al.* Monocrotophos induced oxidative stress and alterations in brain dopamine and serotonin receptors in young rats. Toxicol Ind Health 2016; 32(3): 422-36.
[http://dx.doi.org/10.1177/0748233713500834] [PMID: 24105069]

[52]    Lein PJ, Bonner MR, Farahat FM, *et al.* Experimental strategy for translational studies of organophosphorus pesticide neurotoxicity based on real-world occupational exposures to chlorpyrifos. Neurotoxicology 2012; 33(4): 660-8.
[http://dx.doi.org/10.1016/j.neuro.2011.12.017] [PMID: 22240005]

[53]    Fetoui H, Garoui M, Makni-Ayadi F, Zeghal N. Oxidative stress induced by lambda-cyhalothrin (LTC) in rat erythrocytes and brain: Attenuation by vitamin C. Environ Toxicol Pharmacol 2008; 26(2): 225-31.
[http://dx.doi.org/10.1016/j.etap.2008.04.002] [PMID: 21783916]

[54]    Shafer TJ, Meyer DA, Crofton KM. Developmental neurotoxicity of pyrethroid insecticides: critical review and future research needs. Environ Health Perspect 2005; 113(2): 123-36.
[http://dx.doi.org/10.1289/ehp.7254] [PMID: 15687048]

[55]    Jurisic AD, Petrovic AP, Rajkovic DV, Nicin SDj. The application of lambda-cyhalothrin in tick control. Exp Appl Acarol 2010; 52(1): 101-9.
[http://dx.doi.org/10.1007/s10493-010-9346-z] [PMID: 20309723]

[56]    Kumar A, Rai DK, Sharma B, Pandey RS. Lambda-cyhalothrin and cypermethrin induced *in vivo* alterations in the activity of acetylcholinesterase in a freshwater fish, *Channa punctatus (Bloch)*. Pestic Biochem Physiol 2009; 93: 96-9.
[http://dx.doi.org/10.1016/j.pestbp.2008.12.005]

[57]    Wolansky MJ, Gennings C, Crofton KM. Relative potencies for acute effects of pyrethroids on motor function in rats. Toxicol Sci 2006; 89(1): 271-7.
[http://dx.doi.org/10.1093/toxsci/kfj020] [PMID: 16221961]

[58]    Hossain MM, Richardson JR. Mechanism of pyrethroid pesticide-induced apoptosis: role of calpain and the ER stress pathway. Toxicol Sci 2011; 122(2): 512-25.
[http://dx.doi.org/10.1093/toxsci/kfr111] [PMID: 21555338]

[59]    Narahashi T. Neuronal ion channels as the target sites of insecticides. Pharmacol Toxicol 1996; 79(1): 1-14.
[http://dx.doi.org/10.1111/j.1600-0773.1996.tb00234.x] [PMID: 8841090]

[60]    Takasaki I, Oose K, Otaki Y, *et al.* Type II pyrethroid deltamethrin produces antidepressant-like effects in mice. Behav Brain Res 2013; 257: 182-8.
[http://dx.doi.org/10.1016/j.bbr.2013.09.044] [PMID: 24079995]

[61]    Ansari RW, Shukla RK, Yadav RS, *et al.* Cholinergic dysfunctions and enhanced oxidative stress in the neurobehavioral toxicity of lambda-cyhalothrin in developing rats. Neurotox Res 2012; 22(4): 292-309. a
[http://dx.doi.org/10.1007/s12640-012-9313-z] [PMID: 22327935]

[62]    Ansari RW, Shukla RK, Yadav RS, *et al.* Involvement of dopaminergic and serotonergic systems in the neurobehavioral toxicity of lambda-cyhalothrin in developing rats. Toxicol Lett 2012; 211(1): 1-9. b
[http://dx.doi.org/10.1016/j.toxlet.2012.02.012] [PMID: 22366556]

[63]    Clark JM, Symington SB. Advances in the mode of action of pyrethroids. Top Curr Chem 2012; 314: 49-72.
[http://dx.doi.org/10.1007/128_2011_268] [PMID: 22025067]

[64]    Bradberry SM, Cage SA, Proudfoot AT, Vale JA. Poisoning due to pyrethroids. Toxicol Rev 2005; 24(2): 93-106.
[http://dx.doi.org/10.2165/00139709-200524020-00003] [PMID: 16180929]

[65]    Sheets LP. A consideration of age-dependent differences in susceptibility to organophosphorus and pyrethroid insecticides. Neurotoxicology 2000; 21(1-2): 57-63.
[PMID: 10794385]

[66]    Whyatt RM, Camann DE, Kinney PL, *et al.* Residential pesticide use during pregnancy among a cohort of urban minority women. Environ Health Perspect 2002; 110(5): 507-14.
[http://dx.doi.org/10.1289/ehp.02110507] [PMID: 12003754]

[67]    Berkowitz GS, Obel J, Deych E, *et al.* Exposure to indoor pesticides during pregnancy in a multiethnic, urban cohort. Environ Health Perspect 2003; 111(1): 79-84.
[http://dx.doi.org/10.1289/ehp.5619] [PMID: 12515682]

[68]    Heudorf U, Angerer J, Drexler H. Current internal exposure to pesticides in children and adolescents in Germany: urinary levels of metabolites of pyrethroid and organophosphorus insecticides. Int Arch Occup Environ Health 2004; 77(1): 67-72.
[http://dx.doi.org/10.1007/s00420-003-0470-5] [PMID: 14551781]

[69]    Morgan MK, Sheldon LS, Croghan CW, Jones PA, Chuang JC, Wilson NK. An observational study of 127 preschool children at their homes and daycare centers in Ohio: environmental pathways to cis- and trans-permethrin exposure. Environ Res 2007; 104(2): 266-74.
[http://dx.doi.org/10.1016/j.envres.2006.11.011] [PMID: 17258193]

[70]    Liu CH, Huang CY, Huang CC. Occupational neurotoxic diseases in taiwan. Saf Health Work 2012; 3(4): 257-67.
[http://dx.doi.org/10.5491/SHAW.2012.3.4.257] [PMID: 23251841]

[71]    Grandjean P, Landrigan PJ. Developmental neurotoxicity of industrial chemicals. Lancet 2006; 368(9553): 2167-78.
[http://dx.doi.org/10.1016/S0140-6736(06)69665-7] [PMID: 17174709]

[72]    Debes F, Budtz-Jørgensen E, Weihe P, White RF, Grandjean P. Impact of prenatal methylmercury exposure on neurobehavioral function at age 14 years. Neurotoxicol Teratol 2006; 28(5): 536-47.
[http://dx.doi.org/10.1016/j.ntt.2006.02.005] [PMID: 17067778]

[73]    Szychowski KA, Wójtowicz AK. Components of plastic disrupt the function of the nervous system. Postepy Hig Med Dosw 2013; 67: 499-506.
[http://dx.doi.org/10.5604/17322693.1051001] [PMID: 23752602]

[74]    Woimant F, Trocello JM. Disorders of heavy metals. Handb Clin Neurol 2014; 120: 851-64.
[http://dx.doi.org/10.1016/B978-0-7020-4087-0.00057-7] [PMID: 24365357]

[75]    Caserta D, Graziano A, Lo Monte G, Bordi G, Moscarini M. Heavy metals and placental fetal-maternal barrier: a mini-review on the major concerns. Eur Rev Med Pharmacol Sci 2013; 17(16): 2198-206.
[PMID: 23893187]

[76]    Liu KS, Hao JH, Zeng Y, Dai FC, Gu PQ. Neurotoxicity and biomarkers of lead exposure: a review. Chin Med Sci J 2013; 28(3): 178-88.
[http://dx.doi.org/10.1016/S1001-9294(13)60045-0] [PMID: 24074621]

[77] Jacks G, Bhattacharya P. Arsenic contamination in the environment due to the use of CCAwood preservatives. Arsenic in Wood Preservatives, Part I, Kemi Report 1998; 3: 7-75.

[78] Bhattacharya P, Jacks G, Frisbie SH, *et al.* Arsenic in the Environment: A Global Perspective.Handbook of Heavy Metals in the Environment. New York: Marcell Dekker Inc. 2002; pp. 147-215.
[http://dx.doi.org/10.1201/9780203909300.ch6]

[79] Chiou HY, Huang WI, Su CL, Chang SF, Hsu YH, Chen CJ. Dose-response relationship between prevalence of cerebrovascular disease and ingested inorganic arsenic. Stroke 1997; 28(9): 1717-23.
[http://dx.doi.org/10.1161/01.STR.28.9.1717] [PMID: 9303014]

[80] Rodríguez VM, Carrizales L, Jiménez-Capdeville ME, Dufour L, Giordano M. The effects of sodium arsenite exposure on behavioral parameters in the rat. Brain Res Bull 2001; 55(2): 301-8.
[http://dx.doi.org/10.1016/S0361-9230(01)00477-4] [PMID: 11470331]

[81] Alam MG, Allinson G, Stagnitti F, Tanaka A, Westbrooke M. Arsenic contamination in Bangladesh groundwater: a major environmental and social disaster. Int J Environ Health Res 2002; 12(3): 235-53.
[http://dx.doi.org/10.1080/0960312021000000998] [PMID: 12396524]

[82] Kapaj S, Peterson H, Liber K, Bhattacharya P. Human health effects from chronic arsenic poisoning--a review. J Environ Sci Health A Tox Hazard Subst Environ Eng 2006; 41(10): 2399-428.
[http://dx.doi.org/10.1080/10934520600873571] [PMID: 17018421]

[83] Mukherjee A, Sengupta MK, Hossain MA, *et al.* Arsenic contamination in groundwater: a global perspective with emphasis on the Asian scenario. J Health Popul Nutr 2006; 24(2): 142-63.
[PMID: 17195556]

[84] Brinkel J, Khan MH, Kraemer A. A systematic review of arsenic exposure and its social and mental health effects with special reference to Bangladesh. Int J Environ Res Public Health 2009; 6(5): 1609-19.
[http://dx.doi.org/10.3390/ijerph6051609] [PMID: 19543409]

[85] World Health Organisation (WHO). Arsenic in Drinking-water. Background document for development of WHO Guidelines for Drinking-water Quality. WHO Press, World Health Organization, 20 Avenue Appia, 1211 Geneva 27, Switzerland 2011. WHO/SDE/WSH/ 03.04/75/Rev/1.

[86] Agency for Toxic Substances and Disease Registry (ATSDR). Draft toxicological profile for arsenic. Atlanta, US: US Department of Health and Human Services 2005.

[87] Vahidnia A, van der Straaten RJ, Romijn F, van Pelt J, van der Voet GB, de Wolff FA. Arsenic metabolites affect expression of the neurofilament and tau genes: an *in-vitro* study into the mechanism of arsenic neurotoxicity. Toxicol In Vitro 2007; 21(6): 1104-12.
[http://dx.doi.org/10.1016/j.tiv.2007.04.007] [PMID: 17553662]

[88] Del Razo LM, Garcia-Vargas GG, Garcia-Salcedo J, *et al.* Arsenic levels in cooked food and assessment of adult dietary intake of arsenic in the Region Lagunera, Mexico. Food Chem Toxicol 2002; 40(10): 1423-31.
[http://dx.doi.org/10.1016/S0278-6915(02)00074-1] [PMID: 12387304]

[89] Rahman MM, Mandal BK, Roychowdhury T, *et al.* Arsenic groundwater contamination and suffering of people in North 24- Parganas, one of the nine arsenic affected districts of West Bengal, India: the seven year study report. J Environ Sci Health 2003; 38: 25-59.
[http://dx.doi.org/10.1081/ESE-120016658] [PMID: 12635818]

[90] Chakraborti D, Sengupta MK, Rahman MM, *et al.* Groundwater arsenic contamination and its health effects in the Ganga-Meghna-Brahmaputra plain. J Environ Monit 2004; 6(6): 74N-83N.
[PMID: 15241847]

[91] Huq SMI, Naidu R. Arsenic in groundwater and contamination of the food chain: Bangladesh scenario.Natural arsenic in groundwater: occurrence, remediation and management. Leiden, The

Netherlands: A.A. Balkema 2005; pp. 95-101.

[92]   Järup L, Pershagen G, Wall S. Cumulative arsenic exposure and lung cancer in smelter workers: a dose-response study. Am J Ind Med 1989; 15(1): 31-41.
[http://dx.doi.org/10.1002/ajim.4700150105] [PMID: 2929606]

[93]   Ranft U, Miskovic P, Pesch B, *et al*. Association between arsenic exposure from a coal-burning power plant and urinary arsenic concentrations in Prievidza District, Slovakia. Environ Health Perspect 2003; 111(7): 889-94.
[http://dx.doi.org/10.1289/ehp.5838] [PMID: 12782488]

[94]   Ishinishi N, Tsuchiya K, Vahter M, Fowler BA. Handbook on the Toxicology of Metals. Amsterdam: Elsevier 1986; 1: pp. 43-83.

[95]   Wong O, Whorton MD, Foliart DE, Lowengart R. An ecologic study of skin cancer and environmental arsenic exposure. Int Arch Occup Environ Health 1992; 64(4): 235-41.
[http://dx.doi.org/10.1007/BF00378280] [PMID: 1468791]

[96]   Fairfax RE. Exposure to different metals during the demolition of oil-fired boilers. App occup environ hyg 1993; 8: 151-52.

[97]   Sheehy JW, Jones JH. Assessment of arsenic exposures and controls in gallium arsenide production. Am Ind Hyg Assoc J 1993; 54(2): 61-9.
[http://dx.doi.org/10.1080/15298669391354333] [PMID: 8452098]

[98]   Heaven R, Duncan M, Vukelja SJ. Arsenic intoxication presenting with macrocytosis and peripheral neuropathy, without anemia. Acta Haematol 1994; 92(3): 142-3.
[http://dx.doi.org/10.1159/000204205] [PMID: 7871953]

[99]   Wasserman GA, Liu X, Parvez F, *et al*. Water arsenic exposure and children's intellectual function in Araihazar, Bangladesh. Environ Health Perspect 2004; 112(13): 1329-33.
[http://dx.doi.org/10.1289/ehp.6964] [PMID: 15345348]

[100]  von Ehrenstein OS, Poddar S, Yuan Y, *et al*. Children's intellectual function in relation to arsenic exposure. Epidemiology 2007; 18(1): 44-51.
[http://dx.doi.org/10.1097/01.ede.0000248900.65613.a9] [PMID: 17149142]

[101]  Rosado JL, Ronquillo D, Kordas K, *et al*. Arsenic exposure and cognitive performance in Mexican schoolchildren. Environ Health Perspect 2007; 115(9): 1371-5.
[http://dx.doi.org/10.1289/ehp.9961] [PMID: 17805430]

[102]  Yadav RS, Sankhwar ML, Shukla RK, *et al*. Attenuation of arsenic neurotoxicity by curcumin in rats. Toxicol Appl Pharmacol 2009; 240(3): 367-76.
[http://dx.doi.org/10.1016/j.taap.2009.07.017] [PMID: 19631675]

[103]  Yadav RS, Chandravanshi LP, Shukla RK, *et al*. Neuroprotective efficacy of curcumin in arsenic induced cholinergic dysfunctions in rats. Neurotoxicology 2011; 32(6): 760-8.
[http://dx.doi.org/10.1016/j.neuro.2011.07.004] [PMID: 21839772]

[104]  Chandravanshi LP, Yadav RS, Shukla RK, *et al*. Reversibility of changes in brain cholinergic receptors and acetylcholinesterase activity in rats following early life arsenic exposure. Int J Dev Neurosci 2014; 34: 60-75.
[http://dx.doi.org/10.1016/j.ijdevneu.2014.01.007] [PMID: 24517892]

[105]  Gharibzadeh S, Hoseini SS. Arsenic exposure may be a risk factor for Alzheimer's disease. J Neuropsychiatry Clin Neurosci 2008; 20(4): 501.
[http://dx.doi.org/10.1176/jnp.2008.20.4.501] [PMID: 19196946]

[106]  Tsai SY, Chou HY, The HW, Chen CM, Chen CJ. The effects of chronic arsenic exposure from drinking water on the neurobehavioral development in adolescence. Neurotoxicology 2003; 24(4-5): 747-53.
[http://dx.doi.org/10.1016/S0161-813X(03)00029-9] [PMID: 12900089]

[107] Ratnaike RN. Acute and chronic arsenic toxicity. Postgrad Med J 2003; 79(933): 391-6.
[http://dx.doi.org/10.1136/pmj.79.933.391] [PMID: 12897217]

[108] Kim DS. Occupational safety Health Research Institute looking back Won-Jin rayon accident 20 years. OSH Res Brief 2010; 32: 8-34.

[109] Kim BS, Choi HR, Won CW. Related factors of diagnosis of chronic carbon disulfide poisoning. Korean J Occup Environ Med 1997; 9: 1-11.

[110] Lim Y, Yim HW, Kim KA, Yunm IJ. Review on the manganese poisoning. Korean J Occup Health 1991; 30: 13-8.

[111] Kim EA, Kang SK. Occupational neurological disorders in Korea. J Korean Med Sci 2010; 25 (Suppl.): S26-35.
[http://dx.doi.org/10.3346/jkms.2010.25.S.S26] [PMID: 21258587]

[112] Vyskocil A, Truchon G, Leroux T, *et al.* A weight of evidence approach for the assessment of the ototoxic potential of industrial chemicals. Toxicol Ind Health 2012; 28(9): 796-819.
[http://dx.doi.org/10.1177/0748233711425067] [PMID: 22064681]

[113] Guthrie OW, Xu H, Wong BA, *et al.* Exposure to low levels of jet-propulsion fuel impairs brainstem encoding of stimulus intensity. J Toxicol Environ Health A 2014; 77(5): 261-80.
[http://dx.doi.org/10.1080/15287394.2013.862892] [PMID: 24588226]

[114] Roccisano D, Henneberg M, Saniotis A. A possible cause of Alzheimer's dementia - industrial soy foods. Med Hypotheses 2014; 82(3): 250-4.
[http://dx.doi.org/10.1016/j.mehy.2013.11.033] [PMID: 24440006]

[115] Pattison JE, Bachmann DJ, Beddoe AH. Gamma Dosimetry at Surfaces of Cylindrical Containers. J Radiol Prot 1996; 16: 249-61.
[http://dx.doi.org/10.1088/0952-4746/16/4/004]

[116] Pattison JE. Finger doses received during 153Sm injections. Health Phys 1999; 77(5): 530-5.
[http://dx.doi.org/10.1097/00004032-199911000-00006] [PMID: 10524506]

[117] Motawi TK, Darwish HA, Moustafa YM, Labib MM. Biochemical modifications and neuronal damage in brain of young and adult rats after long-term exposure to mobile phone radiations. Cell Biochem Biophys 2014; 70(2): 845-55.
[http://dx.doi.org/10.1007/s12013-014-9990-8] [PMID: 24801773]

[118] Koivisto M, Krause CM, Revonsuo A, Laine M, Hämäläinen H. The effects of electromagnetic field emitted by GSM phones on working memory. Neuroreport 2000; 11(8): 1641-3.
[http://dx.doi.org/10.1097/00001756-200006050-00009] [PMID: 10852216]

[119] Smythe JW, Costall B. Mobile phone use facilitates memory in male, but not female, subjects. Neuroreport 2003; 14(2): 243-6.
[http://dx.doi.org/10.1097/00001756-200302100-00017] [PMID: 12598738]

[120] Trosic I, Busljeta I, Modlic B. Investigation of the genotoxic effect of microwave irradiation in rat bone marrow cells: *in vivo* exposure. Mutagenesis 2004; 19(5): 361-4.
[http://dx.doi.org/10.1093/mutage/geh042] [PMID: 15388808]

[121] Lee TM, Ho SM, Tsang LY, *et al.* Effect on human attention of exposure to the electromagnetic field emitted by mobile phones. Neuroreport 2001; 12(4): 729-31.
[http://dx.doi.org/10.1097/00001756-200103260-00023] [PMID: 11277573]

[122] Krause CM, Sillanmäki L, Koivisto M, *et al.* Effects of electromagnetic fields emitted by cellular phones on the electroencephalogram during a visual working memory task. Int J Radiat Biol 2000; 76(12): 1659-67. a
[http://dx.doi.org/10.1080/09553000050201154] [PMID: 11133048]

[123] Krause CM, Sillanmäki L, Koivisto M, *et al.* Effects of electromagnetic field emitted by cellular phones on the EEG during a memory task. Neuroreport 2000; 11(4): 761-4. b

[http://dx.doi.org/10.1097/00001756-200003200-00021] [PMID: 10757515]

[124]  Eberhardt JL, Persson BR, Brun AE, Salford LG, Malmgren LO. Blood-brain barrier permeability and nerve cell damage in rat brain 14 and 28 days after exposure to microwaves from GSM mobile phones. Electromagn Biol Med 2008; 27(3): 215-29.
[http://dx.doi.org/10.1080/15368370802344037] [PMID: 18821198]

[125]  Çetin H, Nazıroğlu M, Çelik Ö, Yüksel M, Pastacı N, Özkaya MO. Liver antioxidant stores protect the brain from electromagnetic radiation (900 and 1800 MHz)-induced oxidative stress in rats during pregnancy and the development of offspring. J Matern Fetal Neonatal Med 2014; 27(18): 1915-21.
[http://dx.doi.org/10.3109/14767058.2014.898056] [PMID: 24580725]

[126]  Mehrotra S, Pecaut MJ, Gridley DS. Minocycline modulates cytokine and gene expression profiles in the brain after whole-body exposure to radiation. In Vivo 2014; 28(1): 21-32.
[PMID: 24425832]

[127]  Li X, Wilder-Smith CH, Kan ME, Lu J, Cao Y, Wong RK. Combat-training stress in soldiers increases S100B, a marker of increased blood-brain-barrier permeability, and induces immune activation. Neuroendocrinol Lett 2014; 35(1): 58-63.
[PMID: 24625912]

[128]  National Institute for Occupational Safety and Health (NIOSH). Exposure to stress: Occupational Hazards in Hospitals Department of Health and Human Services, Centers for Disease Control and Prevention, National Institute for Occupational Safety and Health 2008; 136. Available from: www.cdc.gov/niosh/eNews. Publication No. 2008–136

[129]  Bath KG, Schilit A, Lee FS. Stress effects on BDNF expression: effects of age, sex, and form of stress. Neuroscience 2013; 239: 149-56.
[http://dx.doi.org/10.1016/j.neuroscience.2013.01.074] [PMID: 23402850]

[130]  Munakata M. Lifestyle-related disease, stroke and coronary artery disease. Nihon Rinsho 2014; 72(2): 281-7.
[PMID: 24605528]

[131]  Koyama F. Measuring the current status of suicide and depression in workers. Nihon Rinsho 2014; 72(2): 328-32.
[PMID: 24605536]

[132]  Danzer SC. Depression, stress, epilepsy and adult neurogenesis. Exp Neurol 2012; 233(1): 22-32.
[http://dx.doi.org/10.1016/j.expneurol.2011.05.023] [PMID: 21684275]

[133]  Malberg JE, Duman RS. Cell proliferation in adult hippocampus is decreased by inescapable stress: reversal by fluoxetine treatment. Neuropsychopharmacology 2003; 28(9): 1562-71.
[http://dx.doi.org/10.1038/sj.npp.1300234] [PMID: 12838272]

[134]  Borchini R, Ferrario MM. Job strain and heart rate variability. New evidence and new prospects. G Ital Med Lav Ergon 2012; 34(3) (Suppl.): 174-6.
[PMID: 23405612]

[135]  Soleimani SMA, Ekhtiari H, Cadet JL. Drug-induced neurotoxicity in addiction medicine: From prevention to harm reduction. Progress in Brain Research 2016; 223 ISSN 0079-6123
[http://dx.doi.org/10.1016/bs.pbr.2015.07.004]

# CHAPTER 3

# Cancer as an Occupational Hazard

**Manzoor Ahmad Gatoo**[*] and **Sufia Naseem**

*Department of Biochemistry, JN Medical College, AMU, Aligarh, Uttar Pradesh, India*

**Abstract:** Cancer is one of the most dreaded diseases of mankind that causes alarming mortality and morbidity in humans. According to **International Labour Office (ILO)**, Occupational cancer is the most common work-related cause of death, leaving accidents and account for 32% of all work-related deaths worldwide leaving accidents and other occupational diseases well behind. It has long been evident that cancer has a multi-factorial etiology and is a multi-stepped process involving initiation, promotion and tumor progression. Studying occupational cancer is very challenging because of the long latency of cancer and the involvement of many factors in the development of cancer including family history, personal characteristics, dietary and personal habits besides exposure to cancer-causing agents in the workplace and environment. Occupational factors continue to be highly prevalent in new or upgraded IARC (International Agency for Research on Cancer) classifications in last decade. Inhalation, skin exposure and ingestion are significant modes of exposure of chemicals resulting in Cancer.Prevention of occupational cancer is a multistep strategy which involves eradication/minimization of carcinogenic process or agent coupled with good work /hygiene practices, employee education /counselling and workplace monitoring.

**Keywords:** Carcinogen, Chemical Exposure, Workplace, Phase I And II Reactions, Screening test, latency period, Retrospective cohort, risk mapping, body mapping, Engineering and administrative control measures, environmental monitoring, biological monitoring, biological effect monitoring and health surveillance, Good hygiene practices.

## INTRODUCTION

Cancer is one of the most dreaded diseases of mankind that causes alarming mortality and morbidity in humans. It has long been evident that cancer has a multi-factorial etiology and is a multi-stepped process involving initiation, promotion and tumor progression. Chemical carcinogens, physical agents, ionizing radiation, viruses and other agents have all been implicated in cancer initiation and progression. Each different type of cancer may have its own set of

[*] **Corresponding author Manzoor Ahmad Gatoo:** Department of Biochemistry, JN Medical College, AMU, Aligarh, Uttar Pradesh, India; Tel/Fax: 9596448333 & 7456059862; Email: manzbio@gmail.com

**Farhana Zahir (Ed.)**

causes in which many factors play significant roles (Fig. **1**). These factors include family history, personal characteristics, dietary and personal habits and exposure to cancer-causing agents in the workplace and environment. These factors may act together or in sequence to cause cancer and an individual's risk of developing a particular cancer is influenced by combination of these factors.

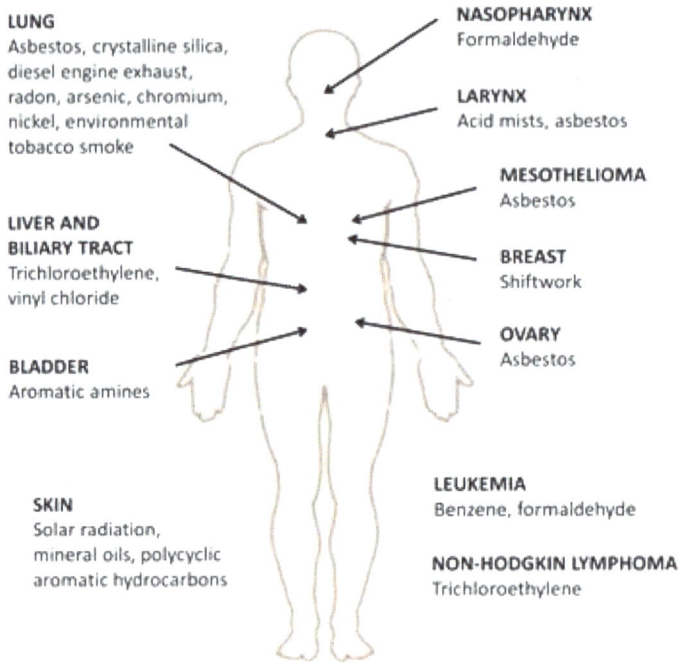

**LUNG**
Asbestos, crystalline silica,
diesel engine exhaust,
radon, arsenic, chromium,
nickel, environmental
tobacco smoke

**LIVER AND
BILIARY TRACT**
Trichloroethylene,
vinyl chloride

**BLADDER**
Aromatic amines

**SKIN**
Solar radiation,
mineral oils, polycyclic
aromatic hydrocarbons

**NASOPHARYNX**
Formaldehyde

**LARYNX**
Acid mists, asbestos

**MESOTHELIOMA**
Asbestos

**BREAST**
Shiftwork

**OVARY**
Asbestos

**LEUKEMIA**
Benzene, formaldehyde

**NON-HODGKIN LYMPHOMA**
Trichloroethylene

**Fig. (1).** Some occupational cancers and workplace exposure.

In 1567, Paracelsus suggested that the 'wasting disease of miners' might be attributed to exposure to realgar (arsenic sulfide) while John Hill reported in 1761 that nasal cancer occurred in some people having habit of using snuff excessively. English surgeon PercivallPott (1744-1788) was the first person to establish a causal link between cancer and exposure to a substance in the workplace. In 1775, he described the occurrence of cancer of scrotum in a number of his male patients, who worked as chimney sweeps in their childhood. He related the malignancy to the occupation of these persons, and concluded that their prolonged workplace exposure to soot was the cause responsible for their malignancy. Pott's description of this disease, and his disquiet for the plight of these 'chimneyboys', sparked a series of reports by other authors and finally resulted in elimination of this practice in England. PercivallPott may be rightly called as a pioneer to the modern investigators who seek to prevent occupational exposure to hazardous substances. Epidemiological studies have played important roles in identification of carcinogenic substances. Rehn (1895) reported an increased prevalence of bladder cancer in aniline dye workers in Germany. The researches have now identified the major carcinogen responsible for cancer in aniline dry workers to be 2-naphthylamine. In early twentieth century, X-ray irradiation was shown to result in skin cancer and sarcoma by Marie Curie, Clunet and Raulot-Lapointe. Yamagiwa and Ichikawa (1915) were the first to induce chemical carcinogenesis in laboratory animals in rabbit model by using coal tar. In 1929, the first pure chemical carcinogen, 1, 2, 5, 6-dibenzanthracene, was synthesized. After that, several chemical carcinogens including polycyclic aromatic hydrocarbons, inorganic compounds and metals have been shown to exhibit carcinogenic properties. The International Agency for Research on Cancer (IARC) Monographs on the Evaluation of Carcinogenic Risks to Humans, provide reviews of occupational exposures and other factors for possible carcinogenicity. From evaluation of IARC Monograph through 2003, it was observed that occupational factors represent 31%, 42%, and 42%, respectively, of factors classified as Sufficient, Probable, and Possible human carcinogens. Occupational factors [1] continue to be highly prevalent in new or upgraded IARC classifications in the last decade. Occupational exposures that have been upgraded include formaldehyde, butadiene, various cobalt & lead compounds and carbon black. Similarly, shift work, which was evaluated for the first time in 2007, has been kept in category of probable human carcinogen while titanium dioxide and talc have been included in the category of possible human carcinogens. Most of the earlier studies related to occupation as risk factor for cancer were done in developed countries [2] but now, studies are also being conducted in developing countries. Studying occupational cancer is very challenging because of the long latency of cancer and the involvement of many factors in its development [3]. **Exposure to more than one potentially cancer causing agents could result in no interaction, an additive effect or more than additive effect.**

Classic human carcinogens first identified in the occupational environment such as arsenic, asbestos, benzene, benzidine, chromium, mustard gas, nickel, radon, and vinyl chloride have established the role of occupation as potential hazard in development of human cancer. Besides these well-established carcinogens, there is a very long list of workplace exposures that are suspected human carcinogens.

The information regarding carcinogenic potential of chemical or physical agents is collected by studies that examine the relationship between an exposure and the risk of developing cancer in human populations/laboratory animals or by tests that evaluate the ability of agent to cause mutations in cells. For identification of carcinogens, several organisations evaluate the available information and categorize the carcinogen in appropriate category. Most authoritative lists of carcinogens are published by IARC (International Agency for Research on Cancer), ACGIH (American Conference of Governmental Industrial Hygienists) and NTP (US National Toxicology Program). IARC, an agency of the World Health Organization, classifies each agent or exposure into one of five groups according to the strength of scientific evidence for carcinogenicity, as follows:

Group 1 - Carcinogenic to humans;
Group 2A - Probably carcinogenic to humans;
Group 2B - Possibly carcinogenic to humans;
Group 3 - Not classifiable as to carcinogenicity to humans and
Group 4 - Probably not carcinogenic to humans

ACGIH, an independent US organization, assigns each chemical or agent to one of the following 5 categories:

A1 - Confirmed human carcinogen;
A2 - Suspected human carcinogen;
A3 - Confirmed animal carcinogen with unknown relevance to humans;
A4 - Not classifiable as a human carcinogen and
A5 - Not suspected as a human carcinogen.

NTP, an interagency programme of US government, publishes a biennial list of agents that they evaluate and assign them to one of the two categories given below.

• Known to be Human Carcinogens
• Reasonably Anticipated to be Human Carcinogens

**Incidence of Occupational Cancer**

According to International Labour Office (ILO), occupational cancer is the most common work-related cause of death which accounts for 32% of all work-related deaths worldwide leaving accidents and other occupational diseases well behind. ILO's cautious estimate puts the cancer toll at over 600,000 deaths a year which means that in every 52 seconds, an individual die due to work related cancer. A World Health Organisation (WHO) study concluded that about 20-30 per cent of males and 5-20 per cent of females of workers could have been exposed to an occupational lung cancer risk during their occupation. A French study conducted by French national statistic office DARES published in 2005 concluded that 13.5 per cent of the total French workforce was exposed to one or more workplace carcinogens which were much higher than estimated a decade earlier. It further concluded that blue collar workers were eight times more at risk than managers. The European Union's CAREX database of occupational exposures to carcinogens estimated that in the early 1990s overall 32 million workers which constituted 23 per cent of the working population had workplace exposures associated with an occupational cancer risk in the then 15 EU member states. The database further concluded that about 95 per cent of causes of lung cancer were identified in workplace studies.

Although studies have been conducted by international and national agencies and organizations to assess the incidence of occupational related cancer, overall impact of occupation on cancer incidence has not been fully evaluated [4] as these studies have been mostly conducted in big cities in industrial workplace and does not take into consideration small industries and small firms. Secondly, new factors and new substances can present new risks and by the time cancers emerge, the substance, process and even the workplace may be long gone. Thirdly, it is a fact that industry finances studies so that risk posed by some occupations is suppressed or played down thus undermining the real threat to humans due to occupational exposure. Fourthly, occupational cancers are usually indistinguishable from cancers which are unrelated to occupation. For example, lung cancer caused by exposure to asbestos is indistinguishable from lung cancer due to tobacco use.

The incidence of cancer related to occupational exposure varies with the type of cancer [5]. The most common types of occupational cancer in United States are lung cancer, bladder cancer and mesothelioma in which percentage of work related cancers is 6.3-13%, 3-19% and 23-90% respectively. Similarly, share of occupational cancer in overall incidence of leukemia, laryngeal, skin cancer, sinonasal/nasopharyngeal cancer, kidney and liver cancer in United States is 0.8-2.8%, 1-20%, 1.5-6%, 31-43%, 0-2.3% and 0.4-1.1% respectively.

## Modes of Exposure

There are three main ways by which workers are exposed to carcinogens at work place and they are inhalation, skin exposure and ingestion.

Inhalation of contaminated air is the most common way through which workplace chemicals enter the body and takes place by breathing of gases, mist, dust, smoke, fumes or vapour containing the hazardous substances. Workplace chemicals enter the air in a number of different ways, evaporation being the most common way by which solids and gases form vapours and enter the air. For example, toluene, methyl ethyl ketone or alcohols enter the air through evaporation. Industrial workplace processes may also generate mists which are formed by gases that condense into small liquid droplets in the air or by breaking up, splashing or atomizing a liquid. For example, acid mists are produced from electroplating while as oil mists are produced from cutting and grinding operations. Other workplace processes can generate dusts, fumes and smoke. Dusts are solid particles often generated by some mechanical or abrasive activity. Fumes are very tiny solid particles generated in welding operations when a heated metal has evaporated in the air and is then condensed back to a solid form. Smoke is carbon or soot produced from burning and depending upon their size, these particles can settle or remain in air. Oxygen in the inhaled breath crosses the alveolar walls to enter the blood within the capillaries for distribution throughout the body. If chemical vapours, gases and mists are present in the inhaled breath, they can reach the alveoli in the lungs and can be passed into the blood for distribution throughout the body. The particulate entry and deposition in the respiratory system depends upon the size, shape and density of the particulate material. Particles are deposited in the lungs by one of four different ways: interception, impaction, sedimentation, and diffusion. During interception, particle travels very near to a surface of the airway passage so that edge of the particle makes contact with the surface leading to deposition of particle. Interception is a common method of deposition by fibres where fibre length decides the place in the airway passage where the particle will be deposited. During impaction, particles do not turn with the air during bend in the airway system but attach to a surface in the particles' original path. Generally, particles having aerodynamic diameter greater than 10 µm are deposited in the nose or throat which prevent them to penetrate deep into respiratory tract. The factors which influence impaction include air velocity and the particle mass. In sedimentation, gravitational force and air resistance overcome buoyancy of particles so that the particle settles on the surface of the lung. Sedimentation is exhibited by particles having aerodynamic diameter of about 0.003 to 5 µm and is most common in the bronchi and the bronchioles. In diffusion, particles are in random motion, which is the main process by which particle deposition in the small airways and alveoli occurs when the speed of the inhaled air has slowed down further. The deposition by diffusion occurs when aerodynamic diameter of particles is less than 0.5 µm.

Skin is the second most common route by which occupational chemicals enter the body. Keratin of epidermis forms a barrier against infections, water, and some chemicals but is much less effective against organic and some inorganic chemicals. Organic and alkaline chemicals can pass through keratin of epidermis to reach the dermis layer, where they are able to enter the veins and then blood stream. In areas of the body having profuse hairs like forearm, chemicals easily penetrate through small ducts containing the hair shaft. Penetration of chemicals can also occur through cuts, punctures or scrapes of the skin and through injection. The extent of penetration of chemicals into the skin varies depending upon their ability to pass through the keratin layer of epidermis. Naptha, toluene and trichloroethylene are unable to penetrate deep in the skin while benzene, carbon tetrachloride, carbon disulfide are able to readily pass through the keratin layer of epidermis. After chemicals penetrate the skin, they are able to get in touch with the blood stream.

Ingestion takes place by swallowing of hazardous substances which occurs through contaminated drinks/food or by swallowing contaminated mucus. After entering the mouth, workplace chemicals pass down into the esophagus and then into the stomach. Most of the chemicals present in contaminated food are transferred from stomach to small intestine which has numerous villi for absorption while some chemicals like alcohol do not move to small intestine and cross the stomach wall to enter into veins and then blood stream directly. The fate of chemicals which reach small intestine depends upon their ability to cross the thin walls of the villi. If they are able to cross the walls of the villi they can enter the blood stream but if they are unable to cross it due to large size or insolubility, they do not enter the blood stream and will remain in the alimentary canal and are passed out through the faeces. Acids and bases if ingested in high concentrations may cause severe burn damage to the digestive system.

There are several factors which influence the carcinogenic potential of a workplace chemical and include route of entry into the body, potency of carcinogen, amount of chemical entering the body, rate of removal from the body and biological variation. Route of entry into body is important factor as some carcinogens will cause cancer only if inhaled and not by skin contact. Amount or dose also plays role in cancer establishment as amount or dose of a chemical entering the body is one of the most important factors which determine whether a chemical will cause cancer or not. In general, higher exposure increases risk of cancer susceptibility. Carcinogenic potency is a measure of the carcinogenic strength of a chemical. Some chemicals that are weak carcinogens require large doses to cause cancer while strong carcinogens require only small doses to cause cancer. Cancer biologists often use animal tests to determine which amount or dose of a certain chemical can lead to cancer. Rate of removal of workplaces' chemicals is significant as many workplace chemicals which enter the body are excreted unchanged while others are broken down and the breakdown products may be more harmful or less harmful than the original chemical which entered the body. Thus, there is less risk of cancer if the body can break down the inhaled/ingested chemical into less toxic products and/or can rapidly remove the chemical from the body. Individual susceptibility is also important and due to genetic makeup, some people are more susceptible to develop cancer than others. Certain personal habits and traits like smoking and drinking add to risk of work related cancer susceptibility.

## Molecular Basis of Occupational Cancer

Cancer is caused by chemical, physical and/or biological agents. Physical agents include ionizing and non-ionizing radiations but are responsible for less than 5% of all cancer in man in the world. The occupational exposure to radiation occurs in workers engaged in manufacturing and distribution of radioactive materials, radioactive waste disposal, nuclear fuel storage, nuclear fuel fabrication as well as in commercial nuclear power reactors and industrial radiographers. IARC has listed the non-ionizing radio frequency radiation from mobile phones, electric power transmission, and other similar sources as a possible carcinogen. Biological agents play some role in certain cancers including leukemia and Burkitt's lymphoma but generally their role is very limited in etiology of cancer. Viruses are a cause of 20% of total cancers in the world. Hepatitis B and C virus for hepatocellular carcinoma [6] is transmitted through blood, thus it is an occupational hazard. Although the primary etiologic agent maybe workplace exposure to virus. Workplace exposure to chemicals like vinyl chloride or aflatoxin besides lifestyle issues like smoking, drinking also add up to aggravate cancer [7]. Chemical agents and substances play major role in etiology of cancer [8] and are responsible for at least 90% of all human cancers.Chemical carcinogens include all chemical substances which can lead to cancer initiation and/or progression and workers of these and allied industries including pesticide production industry are at high risk of occupational cancer. The occupational hazards associated with pesticide production industry are enormous and are observed not only in workers but also in communities living near manufacturing or processing facilities. It has been observed that low income communities working in these units are at major risk of occupational diseases including cancer as they not only work in these industries but also reside near these units. The recent advent of nanotechnology and its widespread applications have led to studies evaluating occupational hazards associated with this emerging field of science. The exposure of workers to nanomaterials having varied shapes, sizes and physico-chemical properties at workplace occurs during manufacturing through principal modes of inhalation, skin contact or ingestion. Although it cannot be concluded that workplace exposure to manufactured nanoparticles **(MNP)** causes cancer, it is likely that occupational hazard associated with manufactured nanomaterials varies depending upon their intrinsic activities and period of exposure. Low toxicity low solubility **(LTLS)** manufactured nanoparticles due to less biological activity are not associated with cancer risk while nanoparticles with more reactive surface may lead to secondary carcinogenesis. It has been observed that **CNT** (carbon nanotubes) can cause genetic aberrations while high aspect ratio nanoparticles **(HARN)** are associated with cancer of lungs, pleural and peritoneal mesothelium. Quartz exposure is associated with silicosis and development of lung cancer while there is sufficient evidence in humans for the carcinogenicity of inhaled crystalline silica in the form of quartz or crystalline silica from occupational sources. Similarly, exposure to asbestos leads to development of lung cancer. Diesel exhaust is a nanoparticle complex containing a mixture of combustion-derived chemicals many of which could be carcinogenic including metals and organic substances.

The experimental animal models have played important role in our understanding of the mechanism of carcinogenesis induced by chemicals at workplace and has helped us to correlate certain occupations/workplace chemical exposure with development of some specific types of cancer. **Epidemiological studies** are usually conducted to detect and correlate occupational exposure with different types of cancer but in these studies, the group which are at high risk of exposure to chemicals is generally small and it is difficult to assess effect of such groups in larger groups of population. Secondly, the epidemiological studies [9] are more valuable in finding the cause of rare or unusual tumors including mesothelioma caused by asbestos and nasal tumors among wood workers *etc.* but are not more effective in detecting normal human cancers.

On the basis of biochemical mode of action, chemical carcinogens can be divided into **direct acting substances** and **procarcinogens** that require metabolic activation. Direct acting substances are chemically reactive substances that act directly on DNA and do not need metabolic transformation. They include alkylating agents, such as mustard gas, ethylene amines, nitrogen mustard and related compounds. Among these mustard gas and bischloromethyl ether are known to cause occupational cancer in man. Some of the most significant targets of alkylating agents such as mustard gas are guanine bases in DNA. The procarcinogens that require metabolic activation include polycyclic and aromatic hydrocarbons, aromatic amines, amides, nitrosamines, natural plant and microbial products *etc.* Fig. (**2A**) depicts the structure of some direct acting occupational carcinogens while Fig. (**2B**) depicts the structure of some occupational carcinogens that require metabolic activation.

When cell is functioning under normal conditions, tightly controlled excitatory and inhibitory pathways regulate cell functioning. Basic cellular functions under these controls include cell division, adhesion, differentiation and senescence. These regulatory pathways are composed of extra cellular ligands which bind to cell-surface receptors to generate intracellular signals sent through secondary messengers. These signals either directly alter cell function or stimulate the transcription of genes whose proteins effect change. Cancer is the outcome of an accumulation of changes in the excitatory and inhibitory cellular pathways and it has been estimated that from three to six somatic mutations are required to transform a normal cell into malignant cell.

### *Direct Acting Agents*

**Mustard Gas**　　　**Butadiene Diepoxide**　　　**Nitrogen Mustards**

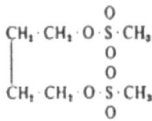

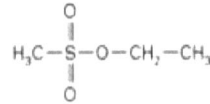

**Dimesyl Glycols Myleran**　　　**β-PropiolactoneEthyl**　　　**Methane Sulphonate**

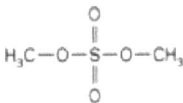

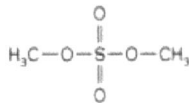

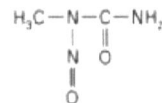

**Dimethyl Sulphate(DMS)**　　　**Nitrogen Mustard**　　　**Methyl Nitrosoureas (MNU)**

**CaproylEthyleneimine**　　　**Dimethyl carbomyl chloride**　　　**Cyclophosphamide**

**Fig. (2A).** Structue of some direct acting carcinogens.

Molecular epidemiological studies have now provided evidence that an individual's susceptibility to occupational cancer [10] is modulated by both genetic [11]. and environmental factors. The environment-gene interaction [12] on chemical carcinogenesis [13] has been well documented by phase-1 and phase-2 enzymes that are involved in the metabolism of carcinogens. The phase I enzymes activate many environmental procarcinogens by adding or exposing their functional groups. Most chemical carcinogens require metabolic activation by phase-1 enzymes and detoxification by phase-2 enzymes. After exposure of humans to chemical carcinogen [14], it may be absorbed in several ways and takes place by means of active or passive transport. The absorption of chemical carcinogen is greatly influenced by physicochemical properties of the substance. The absorption of the substance occurs orally or in the lungs but both of these finally reach liver, the former reaches liver before its distribution by the blood while later reaches liver after their distribution by the blood. Metabolic activation is controlled by phase I reactions, while phase II reactions protect the body through the transformation of activated compounds into inert products which are easily eliminated from the body. Phase I enzymes are involved in metabolic activation of chemical carcinogens and show oxidation, reduction and hydrolysis reactions which finally lead to activation of procarcinogen into carcinogen. Liver is the principal organ where the metabolic activation of pro carcinogens occurs but it can also take place in other organs and organ systems including lungs, kidneys, gastrointestinal system and oesophagus. In the liver, cytochrome P450 is abundant which plays an important role in activation of procarcinogens. The enzymes involved in phase II reactions include transferases and are involved in conjugation and inactivation reactions which detoxify/inactivate the chemical carcinogen. Enzymes of Phase II reactions are mainly involved in conjugation reactions leading to formation of less toxic metabolites which are more water soluble and are more readily excreted from the body.

*Indirect Acting Agents:*

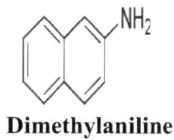

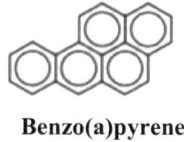

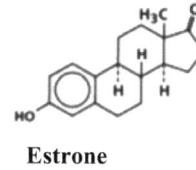

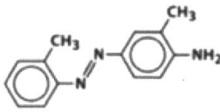

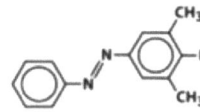

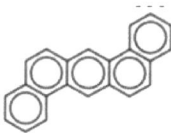

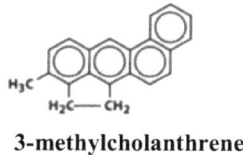

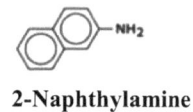

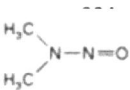

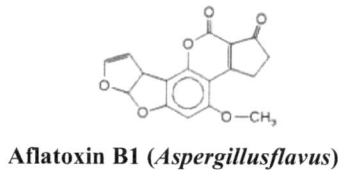

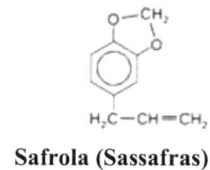

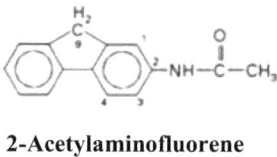

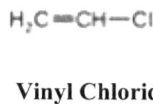

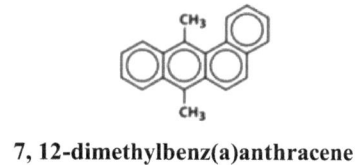

Dimethylaniline                Benzo(a)pyrene                Estrone

2,3-Dimethyl-4-amino-azobenzene            N,N-Dimethyl-4-aminoazobenzene

Dibenz(a,h)anthracene        3-methylcholanthrene        2-Naphthylamine

Dimethylnitrosamine    Aflatoxin B1 (*Aspergillusflavus*)    Safrola (Sassafras)

2-Acetylaminofluorene        Vinyl Chloride        7, 12-dimethylbenz(a)anthracene

**Fig. (2B).** Structure of some indirect acting workplace carcinogens that reqire metabolic activation.

Thus the coordinated expression and regulation of phase-1 and phase-2 xenobiotic metabolizing enzymes and their metabolic balance may be an important factor in determining whether exposure to carcinogen results in cancer or not. The exposure to chemical carcinogens at workplace can result in damage of DNA, which if left unrepaired, could lead to the process of carcinogenesis. To safeguard the integrity of genome, humans have developed a set of complex DNA repair systems. The major pathways of DNA repair include base excision repair, nucleotide excision repair and double strand break repair. Base excision repair pathway repairs minor base alterations such as oxidized or reduced bases or methylated bases while nucleotide excision repair pathway repairs bulky lesions such as pyrimidine dimers, large chemical adducts. Double strand break repair (DSB) is done by homologous/non homologous pathway. Because of the importance of maintaining genomic integrity in the general and specialized functions of cell as well as in prevention of carcinogens, genes coding for DNA repair molecules have been proposed as candidate cancer susceptibility genes.

Genetic damage [15] due to mutations in cancer cells can be divided into two categories, dominant and recessive changes. Dominant changes, most frequently occur in proto-oncogenes but can also occur in certain tumor suppressor genes and result in gain of function. Recessive mutations occur most commonly in growth-inhibitory pathway genes and tumor suppressor genes and result in loss of gene function. Oncogenes play an important role in the initiation and progression of neoplasia. Aberrant expression of the proto-oncogenes, epidermal growth factor receptor (EGFR)/c-erb 1, members of the ras family, as well as c-myc is an important role in development and progression of cancer. Intracellular messengers can also be intrinsically activated leading to their continuous activation even in the absence of ligand whereas in normal conditions, they become inactive in the absence of ligand. Overexpression of transcriptional factors like C-myc, C-raf and C-junetc. has been observed to be associated with the development of cancer. Tumor suppressor genes act as strong negative regulatory controls of cancer which are inactivated during tumor formation due to chromosomal alterations. Loss of activity of tumor suppressor genes is considered a major event in the pathway of carcinogenesis leading to the development of cancer. Tumor suppressor genes, unlike oncogenes, need inactivation of both the copies of genes by deletions, rearrangements, point mutations *etc.* while oncogenes require activation of only one of the two gene copies for their activity. p53, the product of tumor suppressor gene TP53 and localized on 17p 13.1, has a central role in the control of the cell cycle of cells bearing sub lethal damage within their genome. It arrests the cell cycle in the late G1 phase until repair of the genomic damage or causes induction of apoptosis. On one hand, activation of proto oncogenes undermines the regulatory pathways of cell cycle leading to growth promotion while on other hand, inactivation of tumor suppressor genes allows cell to evade growth-inhibitory pathways. These events can occur at any level of the growth-inhibitory signal transduction pathway. Thus mutations caused by DNA damage can lead to activation of proto oncogenes, inactivation of tumor suppressor genes and/or alteration of cell cycle regulator genes which leads to expression of altered gene products and loss of regulatory genes. Afterwards, invasion and metastasis occurs in precancerous cell for transformation into malignant cell. Fig. (**3**) depicts the molecular basis of process of carcinogenesis.

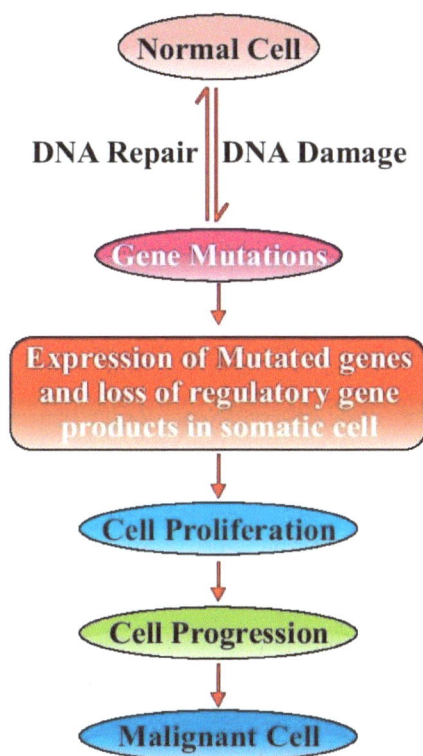

**Fig. (3).** Molecular Basis of Cancer.

Some scientists have classified chemical carcinogens on the basis of their mechanism of action into genotoxic example nickel chloride and non genotoxic carcinogens example arsenic. Genotoxic carcinogens are direct acting substances which alter genetic information of cell both quantitatively and qualitatively. They are active in high doses leading to cell toxicity and increase in cell proliferation and DNA replication. Genotoxic carcinogens interact directly with DNA, RNA and proteins changing their structural integrity and lead to formation of adducts which represent the first decisive step towards carcinogenesis which if left unrepaired before DNA replication lead to mutation in proto-oncogenes and tumor suppressor genes which are primary events in the initiation of carcinogenesis. Mutations linked to adduct can appear through deletion, frameshift, or by nucleotide substitution. Various techniques used for identification and analysis of adducts include radioimmunoassay, fluorescent and mass spectrometry techniques. Non genotoxic carcinogens do not react directly with DNA and do not need metabolic activation but act as promoters which modulate growth and cell death whose exposure favours the synthesis of other substances responsible for neoplastic development. They do not form adducts and show negative mutagenicity tests both *in vitro* and *in vivo*. Non genotoxic carcinogens may function as tumorpromotors, endocrine modifiers, receptor mediator or immunosuppressants. Chemical carcinogens can have additional synergic or antagonistic effects when simultaneously presented in different metabolic ways which is evident from increased incidence of lung cancer in those workers which are exposed to asbestos and also have smoking habit.

Initiation is the first stage of carcinogenesis which is caused by irreversible genetic changes and predisposes normal cells towards malignancy and these genetic changes are transmitted to daughter cells. In the initiated cell, mutations occur that induce proliferation which is essential for this stage. The main event in initiation is DNA damage and formation of DNA adducts. Initiation process is affected by dose of carcinogen and with increase in dose, the incidence of cancer increases. Initiation can be both spontaneous and induced but frequency of spontaneous initiation is very low as DNA repair systems have in built capacity to prevent any such process from transformation into malignant neoplasm.

During promotion stage, promoter compounds do not interact directly with DNA but can indirectly damage DNA as well as increase cell proliferation in susceptible tissues, increase variations in genetic expression and cause alteration in pathways that control cell growth. The concentration of the promoter determines its effectiveness and it must be present for sufficient time to be effective. The most important activity of promoters is mitogenesis. Promoter agent may be specific for one tissue or may be non-specific acting on numerous tissues. Promotion is a reversible stage that can be moulded up by physiological factors and is referred to as pre-neoplastic stage/benign neoplastic in histopathology.

Progression is the last stage of carcinogenesis which is irreversible stage during which transformation into malign lesions takes place. In progression, a neoplastic phenotype is attained through genetic and epigenetic mechanisms for which angiogenesis must occur. During progression, not only phenotypic changes occur in the cell but it also shows invasion and metastasis which are essential for neoplastic development. Fig. (**4**) depicts different stages of chemical carcinogenesis.

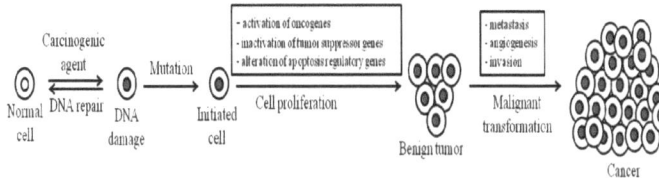

**Fig. (4).** Stages of chemical carcinogenesis.

## Agents Causing Occupational Cancer

The recognition of role of occupation in development of cancer dates back to 1775 when Percival Pott in 1775 reported increased incidence of carcinoma of the scrotum among young chimney sweeps. It is more common to detect unusual tumor at the workplace due to exposure to particular carcinogen like mesothelioma in asbestos workers, bladder cancer in dye workers and angiosarcoma of the liver in vinyl chloride workers. The most affected industries in which there is high incidence of occupational cancer include rubber industry, painting industry and petrochemical related industry. Table **1** gives information about various chemical/physical agents which are known causes of occupational cancer [16].

**Table 1. Various chemical/physical agents which are known causes of occupational cancer.**

| Chemical/ Physical Agent | Cancer (S) |
|---|---|
| Aflatoxin B1 | Liver |
| Alkylating agents | Bladder, leukemia |
| 4-Aminobiphenyl | Bladder |
| Arsenic and Inorganic Arsenic Compounds | Skin, lung, gastro intestinal, kidney |
| Asbestos | Lung, larynx, gastrointestinal, mesothelioma |
| Betel Nut | Buccal mucosa |
| Benzene | Leukemia |
| Benzidine and dyes metabolized to benzidine | Bladder |
| Benzopyrene | Skin, lung, stomach |
| Beryllium and Beryllium Compounds | Lung |
| Cadmium and Cadmium Compounds | Lung |
| Cigarette Smoke | Lung |
| Coke oven emissions | Lung, genitourinary system |
| p-ChloroToulidine | Bladder |
| Chromium Hexavalent Compounds | Lung |

| Chemical/ Physical Agent | Cancer (S) |
|---|---|
| Coal Tars and Coal-Tar Pitches | Skin, lung |
| Ethylene oxide | Leukemia, Lymphatic system, Haemopoetic system |
| Environmental tobacco smoke | Lung |
| Formaldehyde | nasal, pharyngeal, Leukemia |
| Mustard gas | Respiratory tract |
| Mineral Oils (untreated/ mildly refined) | Skin, lung |
| Nickel Compounds | Lung, nasal |
| 2-Napthylamine | Bladder |
| n-Nitrosodimethylamine | Liver, Lungs and Kidney |
| Radon and its decay products | Lung |
| Radiations | Leukemia, Skin, Melanoma |
| Silica | Lung |
| Soot | Lung, skin |
| Vinyl chloride | Liver, brain, lung, lymphatic system, Haemopoetic system |
| Wood dust | Nasal |

## Detection of Cancer in the Workplace

Detection of occupational cancers is one of the real challenges in the field of occupational health due to difficulties in relating exposure at workplace to cancer incidence. The exposure-response relationship has not been properly evaluated in most of the studies which have investigated the relation of workplace exposure to cancer incidence. Besides, very less work has been done on categorizing workplace exposure by type, duration and intensity.

Induction periods of most malignant cancers caused by occupational exposures can vary from 12 to 50 years. During this long induction period, there may have been many changes in the working environment and the worker may not be able to remember all the processes and materials. Job mobility is another factor which makes it difficult to estimate workplace exposure as the worker may have had several jobs in several locations during the induction period and the variation in exposure level in these jobs and locations will compound the difficulty in calculating overall workplace exposure. Confounders and competing risk make estimation of workplace exposure further difficult. As smoking habits, diet, pollution, stress, physical activity and drugs *etc.* have role in incidence of cancer, so evaluation of these factors must be taken into account while estimating the relationship of workplace exposure with cancer so that adjustment for these factors can be made to give real insight about effects of workplace exposure.

By cluster studies, one can detect rare or unusual tumor occurring at workplace but it is not possible to detect common tumors by this approach. For detection of common cancers at workplace, population approach is used. Exposure of a large population to carcinogenic substances might increase the risk of cancer incidence but information regarding specific exposure within the population will lead to identification of subpopulation which will be at higher risk for specific tumors. This has been substantiated by various studies including a large cohort study in rubber workers where population at large did not show any increased incidence of any cancer but after stratification of workers in the departments in which they worked, increased incidence of colon and stomach cancer was observed in workers from rubber-compounding area while workers from the tire-curing area showed increased incidence of lung cancer.

Three principal approaches used to study high risk populations which are exposed to workplace carcinogenic agents include cohort, case-control and proportional mortality study approaches. In **cohort study**, a population that has been exposed to a particular substance/s is followed and the number of tumors that develop as effect of this exposure is determined. This approach allows health professionals to correlate exposure of particular substance/s with various health factors including cancer. **Retrospective cohort** studies are used for identification of single agents whose workplace exposure can lead to malignancy and require large time period to demonstrate that a particular agent is an occupational carcinogen which is done by evaluation of cancer incidence and / or cancer mortality in that population over a long period of time. Examples of agents for which epidemiologic studies provide evidence of an exposure-response relationship include asbestos, benzene, ortho-toluidine, aniline and vinyl chloride *etc.* Vinyl chloride and bischloromethyl ether (BCME) are examples of associations between single agents and rare histological types of cancer. The demonstration of single agent as causative factor for occupational cancer facilitates prevention of such cancers as such agents can be effectively controlled. The findings of such studies are used to assess the effect of decreasing exposure level on cancer incidence and to find out minimum level of carcinogen which can be allowed at workplace. Majority of chemical carcinogens whose exposure level is monitored by different national and international organisations are single- agent exposures.

In **case control study**, patients with specific tumor called cases are compared with normal persons from population which are called **controls**. The presence of tumor in cases is correlated with specific workplace exposure in these patients and exposure of specific carcinogen/s is determined to assess the association of workplace exposure with the incidence of cancer. In proportional mortality study, cause of death as recorded in death certificate is compared with the expected proportions of mortality based on age, race, sex and time of death but one should have access to the death certificates on a group of workers with known exposure. Thus workers who are at high risk of work related cancer are readily recognized by surveillance and case-control studies and may in addition be recognized by cohort studies of workers engaged in those occupations which are at high risk of exposure.

The measurement of hazardous materials in the workplace environment is done by workplace exposure assessment through area sampling or personal sampling. Both methods have their uses, depending on the work conditions and worker mobility. Surveillance is one of the main features for the early detection of occupational cancer and may include risk mapping, body mapping and surveys. In **risk mapping**, basic map of the workplace is drawn while machines, workstations and the substances or processes used at workplace are marked. Documentation of any health problem reported by workers doing particular jobs is done on risk map and this is repeated periodically to arrive at any conclusion. In **body mapping**, workers are asked to mark areas of body having symptom of any disease or having excessive pain. The body mapping can be used to identify effect of exposure of a chemical on workers engaged in particular work within the workplace. For example, if workers doing similar job within the workplace report similar symptoms, then it can be concluded that these symptoms are caused by exposure of that chemical. Besides regular surveys can be done to assess the apprehensions and concerns about a particular job or substance and such survey should also include retired workers as occupational cancer has long induction period.

Workers exposed to chemicals may be monitored using several methods including environmental monitoring, biological monitoring, biological effect monitoring and health surveillance. **Environmental monitoring** is done usually in the form of air sampling and analysis but may include measurement of chemicals on surfaces, clothing, equipment and any other point where the chemical may come in contact with the worker but environmental monitoring does not give direct assessment of *in vivo* exposure of the worker but gives an idea about the contamination of the overall workplace atmosphere so molecular monitoring is used as supplementary tool. In **biological monitoring,** measurement of chemicals or their metabolites in tissues or fluids, such as urine and blood is done which assimilate exposure by all routes and over time and gives an estimate of the overall uptake of chemical by workers at workplace. The main aim of biological monitoring is to assess whether significant uptake has taken place in the workers and is not done for prognostic purposes. For urine analysis, the standardisation for urine volume must be done to arrive at right conclusion about workplace exposure of carcinogen. Creatinine concentration which is indicator of urine dilution can be used to standardise urine volume. It is recommended to record the time of last exposure before sample collection as well as early testing of collected urine sample as some chemical carcinogens including MOCA 4, 4' methylene bis have very short life time and will disappear if urine analysis is done after long time although they may be present at high concentrations in the urine sample initially. Table **2** gives information about measurement of uptake of some occupational carcinogens using urine/blood analysis.

**Table 2. Measurement of Uptake of Some Occupational Carcinogens.**

| Urine Analysis | | |
|---|---|---|
| **Chemical agent** | **Determinant** | **Reference value** |
| Aniline | Total p- Aminophenol | 50 mg/g creatinine |
| Arsenic and inorganic compounds | Inorganic Arsenic metabolites | 50 µ g/g creatinine |
| Benzene | Phenol | 50 mg/g creatinine |
| Cadmium and inorganic compounds | Cadmium | 5 µ g/g creatinine |
| Chlorobenzene | 4-Chlorocathechol<br>p-Chlorophenol | 150 mg/g creatinine<br>25 mg/g creatinine |
| Chromium (V1) | Chromium | 30 mg/g creatinine |
| **Blood Analysis** | | |
| Aniline | Methaemoglobin | 1.5% |
| Cadmium and inorganic compounds | Cadmium | 5 µ g/liter |
| Nitrobenzene | Methaemoglobin | 1.5% |

**Biological effect monitoring** involves the measurement of end-points of biological processes (biochemical, physiological and others) that could be affected by exposure of chemicals and may not be involved in disease occurrence and prognosis. In biological effect monitoring, there is monitoring of interaction of carcinogen with the DNA and any structural change induced by carcinogen exposure [17, 18]. Structural changes in DNA will include DNA strand breaks, chromosomal aberrations, sister chromatid exchanges and loss of heterozygosity. The precancerous stage can be identified by presence of erythroplakia and dysplastic lesions. It is now possible to monitor various stages of cancer from its initial stage of carcinogen exposure to last stage of cancer development which can be of prime importance in early detection of occupational cancer. Fig. (**5**) gives information about different methods of monitoring workers who are at high risk of exposure to occupational carcinogens.

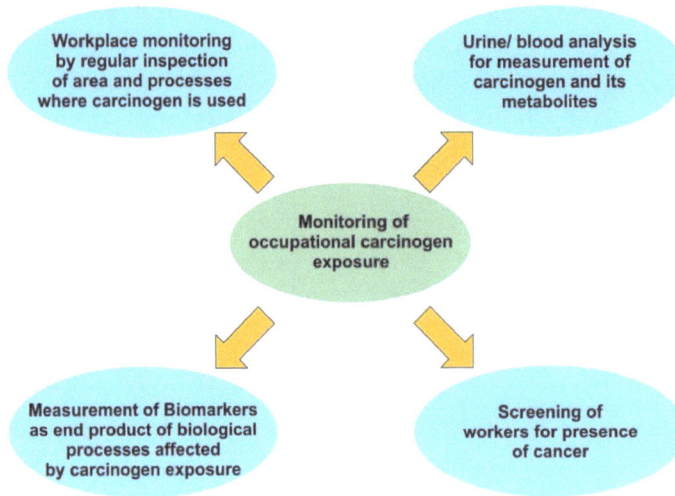

**Fig. (5).** Different methods of monitoring of occupational carcinogen exposure.

**Occupational cancers have long latency periods and in most of cases are not at an early stage when diagnosable symptoms become noticeable.** If these tumors are detected early by ensuing diagnosis at the earliest possible stage, it will increase chances of successful tumor treatment. Classical methods of early diagnosis usually fail to identify the development of new cancer at a very early stage leading to difficulties in treatment of cancer. **Screening test** should be able to identify persons who have or possess high risk of developing cancer due to workplace exposure so that treatment of such persons can be started at the earliest. For example, urine dipstick test is useful for identification of haematuria in workers exposed to aromatic amines which may lead to bladder cancer. Identification of such workers will help in further surveillance and monitoring of these workers so that workplace cancer can be prevented in them. Another important aspect regarding screening programme is that it should continue even after period of actual exposure as occupational cancer have long latency period and may take years to develop. Besides screening of workers should be done periodically and should include not only active workers but also retired employees as occupational cancer usually manifests itself after long latency period.

Various clinical screening tools which are being used for screening subjects at risk of occupational related cancer includeX-ray, spiral CT scanning, sputum cytology, chest x-ray, HRCT scan and urine cytology which are used to detect various cancers in workers exposed to carcinogens. As it is not advised to use CT scan regularly so this screening tool should be used when needed and not on routine basis. Thus, there is urgent need to focus on development of more novel molecular markers which can detect cancer at its early stage. Further these markers need to be validated so that they can be used at large scale. Table **3** gives information about various screening tests for subjects who are at high risk of occupational cancer. **Recently a team of researchers at UNIST (Ulsan National Institute of Technology, South Korea) have introduced a new technique that validates urine biomarker for early detection of cancer and may be useful in clinical settings to test urinary EV based biomarker for early cancer detection. Similarly, Scientists at John Hopkins Kimmel Cancer Centre, USA have discovered a new blood test which has potential to identify eight cancer types (Lung, breast, colorectal, ovarian, liver, stomach, pancreas and esophagus) from one blood sample and may prove to be very useful for early detection of cancer in high risk subjects including those exposed to workplace carcinogens [19].**

Table 3. Clinical screening tests for workers exposed to carcinogens.

| Cancer Type | Screening Test |
| --- | --- |
| Skin Cancer | Skin Examination<br>Skin Biopsy (Shave, Punch, Incision, Excision) |
| Lung Cancer | Chest X-Ray<br>CT Scan<br>Sputum Cytology<br>Spiral CT Scan |
| Bladder Cancer | Cytoscopy<br>Urine Cytology<br>Hematuria |
| Liver Cancer | Serum Tumor Marker (Alpha fetoprotein)<br>Liver Function Test<br>CT Scan<br>MRI<br>Biopsy (FNAC, Core needle, Laparoscopy) |
| Head and Neck Cancers | Throat Examination<br>CT Scan<br>PET Scan<br>MRI<br>Bronchoscopy<br>Endoscopy<br>Esophagoscopy |

## Prevention of Occupational Cancer

As occupational cancers arise as a direct consequence of human activity so ideally all such cancers should be preventable [20]. But keeping in view importance of industrial and other practices for human development, it is not possible to eradicate the source of these cancers but efforts can be directed to minimize and/ or reduce the exposure of these carcinogenic agents at workplace [21]. The aim of preventive strategies is to prevent workers from exposure of any substance/s, processes and environment in the workplace which can increase risk of cancer in the workers. Prevention of occupational cancer is easier than cancers caused due to lifestyle factors like excessive smoking or alcohol intake as occupational cancer can be more easily controlled by preventing exposure of carcinogen.

The most efficient approach for prevention of occupational cancer will include **premarket testing** of all new chemical compounds and industrial processes but premarket testing is not done in most of such cases. Second approach is to take practical measures to control toxic exposures in the workplace by eradication/ minimizing exposure of carcinogens at workplace. Ideally the carcinogenic agent at workplace should be eliminated from the workplace by using alternative agent or technology but elimination of chemical carcinogen or process producing such carcinogens is not feasible in most of cases so efforts should be aimed at minimizing exposure of workers from such agents/ processes at workplace. Besides elimination of such carcinogenic agents/ processes usually require government approval. During installation of industrial plants, it must be ensured that those techniques and processes are employed which minimize the exposure of carcinogenic substances and processes so that workers are prevented from such exposure. Besides it is recommended that such measures be taken for elimination/ reduction of workplace exposure which does not need active support of workers as workers may respond differently to such measures. Measures used to minimise exposure at workplace should be directed at minimizing duration and concentration of exposure as well as decrease in number of persons who are exposed to such agents and processes.

Various methods of controlling worker exposure to chemicals include control at engineering level, administrative level and personal safety equipment. Engineering control measures include isolation of source of exposure, enclosure of area of exposure, availability of exhaust ventilation facilities and modification of process/equipment for reduction of exposure level. Administrative level measures include good work and hygiene practices, high-quality housekeeping, worker education and counselling. Thus exposure of carcinogen can be minimized by isolation of the agent or process, minimizing the number of potentially exposed workers, minimizing the time of potential exposure, reducing the average intensity of exposure, proper work practices, personal protective equipment, personal hygiene, worker education and counselling and workplace monitoring. Isolation means separating the process so that workers who are not directly engaged with that process are prevented from exposure of such process. Isolation usually includes exclusion of that process under enclosed conditions. The number of workers exposed should be minimised without increasing the average exposure of each individual worker which will lead to decline in number of cancer incidence in workers. This can be achieved by several means including restriction in accessibility to such facility to only those personnel who are directly involved in the process involving carcinogenic exposure. The time of expected exposure can be minimized by allowing workers to enter the specified area only when it is indispensable. The average intensity of exposure is reduced by installation of dedicated exhaust systems and personal protective equipment. Proper care must be given to repair and maintenance procedures of carcinogenic processes/ systems. For example, in the manufacture of polyvinyl chloride from vinyl chloride monomer, although the manufacturing is being done under full enclosure but earlier cleaning processes were not automated which resulted in substantial exposure of workers engaged in maintenance of these vessels.

The aim of workplace monitoring is to minimize exposure of workers at workplace by minimizing exposure caused through inhalation, skin contact or oral route. It includes inspection of areas and processes where carcinogen is utilized to check proper functioning of control systems, quantitative measurements of airborne levels of potential carcinogens and their products, regular testing of personal protective equipment for efficiency and suitability, encouragement of good work practices and hygiene practices and measurement of valid biological indexes of exposure. The education of workers which are at risk of exposure to carcinogens is also important in preventing occupational cancer. The workers should be educated about identity and location of different substances at workplace and the hazards associated with these substances including ways of exposure of these substances. The employers should discourage smoking at workplace as it increases the risk of cancer incidence. Workers can be trained to work at places of high exposure so that safe work procedures are adopted.

There should be pre-placement screening of high risk individuals as some non-occupational factors can enhance the risk of occupational cancer. It has been observed that smoking increases the risk of lung cancer in workers who are exposed to asbestos or who inhale radioactive dust. Thus occupational lung cancer can be minimized by placement of individuals who are non-smokers or have long since quit smoking to work in such locations. The workers who have been exposed to carcinogen in the past should be managed in efficient manner. They should not be exposed to carcinogens anymore and should be prohibited from smoking strictly if they are exposed to lung and bladder carcinogens. Dietary modifications may be considered to reduce the likelihood of cancer and screening of such workers can be done to detect pre-clinical cancer or pre-cancerous lesions. Good hygiene practices should be maintained at workplace and workers should be encouraged to use good health and hygiene practices including no tobacco use at workplace, washing of hands before eating/ drinking and avoiding skin contact with chemicals at workplace. **Thus prevention of occupational cancer is a multistep strategy which involves eradication/minimization of carcinogenic process or agent coupled with good work /hygiene practices, employee education /counselling and workplace monitoring.**

## CONSENT FOR PUBLICATION

Not applicable.

## ACKNOWLEDGEMENTS

The authors acknowledge the support and cooperation of Dr. Yair Arafat, Department of Biochemistry, Jawaharlal Nehru Medical College, AMU, Aligarh in writing this manuscript.

## CONFLICT OF INTEREST

The authors confirm that this chapter contents have no conflict of interest.

## REFERENCES

[1]     1. Steenland K, Burnett C, Lalich N, Ward E, Hurrell J. Dying for work:The magnitude of US mortality from selected causes of death associated with occupation. Am J Ind Med 2003 May; 43(5): 461-82.

[2]     Ames BN. The detection of environmental mutagens and potential carcinogens. Cancer 1984; 53(10): 2034-40.
[http://dx.doi.org/10.1002/1097-0142(19840515)53:10<2034::AID-CNCR2820531005>3.0.CO;2-S] [PMID: 6367933]

[3]     Barrett JC. Mechanisms of multistep carcinogenesis and carcinogen risk assessment. Environ Health Perspect 1993; 100: 9-20.
[http://dx.doi.org/10.1289/ehp.931009] [PMID: 8354184]

[4]     Purdue MP, Hutchings SJ, Rushton L, Silverman DT. The proportion of cancer attributable to occupational exposures. Ann Epidemiol 2015; 25(3): 188-92.
[http://dx.doi.org/10.1016/j.annepidem.2014.11.009] [PMID: 25487971]

[5]     Labrèche F, Duguay P, Boucher A, Arcand R. But other than mesothelioma? An estimate of the proportion of work-related cancers in Quebec. Curr Oncol 2016; 23(2): e144-9.
[http://dx.doi.org/10.3747/co.23.2812] [PMID: 27122983]

[6]     Kim H, Chung YK, Kim I. 2018; Recognition criteria for occupational cancers in relation to hepatitis B virus and hepatitis C virus in Korea. Ann Occup Environ Med 30: 6.
[http://dx.doi.org/10.1186/s40557-018-0217-0]

[7]     Santella RM, Wu HC. Environmental Exposures and Hepatocellular Carcinoma. J Clin Transl Hepatol 2013; 1(2): 138-43.
[PMID: 26357611]

[8]     Guengerich FP. Metabolism of chemical carcinogens. Carcinogenesis 2000; 21(3): 345-51.
[http://dx.doi.org/10.1093/carcin/21.3.345] [PMID: 10688854]

[9]     Checkoway H, Pearce NE. Crawford-Brown DJ: Research methods in occupational epidemiology. New York: Oxford University Press 1989.

[10]    Luch A. Nature and nurture - lessons from chemical carcinogenesis. Nat Rev Cancer 2005; 5(2): 113-25.
[http://dx.doi.org/10.1038/nrc1546] [PMID: 15660110]

[11]    Kinzler KW, Vogelstein B. Cancer-susceptibility genes. Gatekeepers and caretakers. Nature 1997; 386(6627): 761-763, 763.
[http://dx.doi.org/10.1038/386761a0] [PMID: 9126728]

[12]    Dixon K, Kopras E. Genetic alterations and DNA repair in human carcinogenesis. Semin Cancer Biol 2004; 14(6): 441-8.
[http://dx.doi.org/10.1016/j.semcancer.2004.06.007] [PMID: 15489137]

[13]    Klaunig JE, Kamendulis LM, Xu Y. Epigenetic mechanisms of chemical carcinogenesis. Hum Exp Toxicol 2000; 19(10): 543-55.
[http://dx.doi.org/10.1191/096032700701546442] [PMID: 11211991]

[14]    Oliveira PA, Colaço A, Chaves R, Guedes-Pinto H, De-La-Cruz P LF, Lopes C. 2007 Dec; Chemical carcinogenesis. An Acad Bras Cienc 79(4): 593-616.
[http://dx.doi.org/10.1590/S0001-37652007000400004]

[15]    Phillips DH, Arlt VM. Genotoxicity: damage to DNA and its consequencesEXS 2009; 99: 87-110.

[16]    Siemiatycki J, Richardson L, Straif K, *et al.* Listing occupational carcinogens. Environ Health Perspect 2004; 112(15): 1447-59.
[http://dx.doi.org/10.1289/ehp.7047] [PMID: 15531427]

[17]    Baird WM, Mahadevan B. The uses of carcinogen- DNA adduct measurement in establishing mechanisms of mutagenesis and in chemoprevention. Mutat Res 2004; 547(13): 1-4.

[18]    Santella RM, Gammon M, Terry M, *et al.* DNA adducts, DNA repair genotype/phenotype and cancer risk. Mutat Res 2005; 592(1-2): 29-35.
[http://dx.doi.org/10.1016/j.mrfmmm.2005.06.001] [PMID: 16023682]

[19]    Cohen JD, Li L, Wang Y, *et al.* Detection and localization of surgically resectable cancers with a multi-analyte blood test. Science 2018; 359(6378): 926-30.
[http://dx.doi.org/10.1126/science.aar3247] [PMID: 29348365]

[20]    Carey RN, Hutchings SJ, Rushton L, *et al.* The future excess fraction of occupational cancer among those exposed to carcinogens at work in Australia in 2012. Cancer Epidemiol 2017; 47: 1-6.
[http://dx.doi.org/10.1016/j.canep.2016.12.009] [PMID: 28081474]

[21]    Landrigan PJ. The prevention of occupational cancer. CA Cancer J Clin 1996; 46(2): 67-9.
[http://dx.doi.org/10.3322/canjclin.46.2.67] [PMID: 8624798]

# CHAPTER 4

# Occupational Health Hazards to Medical and Paramedical Staff

Farhana Zahir[1,*], Shazia Parveen[2], Nasreen Noor[2], Abdul Faiz Faizy[3], Shaziya Allarakha[3] and Shagufta Moin[3]

[1] *Prism Educational Society, Aligarh, Uttar Pradesh, India*

[2] *Department of Obstetrics and Gynaecology, JN Medical College, Aligarh Muslim University, Aligarh, Uttar Pradesh, India*

[3] *Department of Biochemistry, JN Medical College, Aligarh Muslim University, Aligarh, Uttar Pradesh, India*

**Abstract:** In order to deliver quality health care to the community and experience medicine as rewarding career, professionals in healthcare sector also need to be healthy. According to International Labour Organisation (ILO)/World Health Organisation (WHO) declaration on health services 2005, Health care workers are all persons involved in actions whose main intent is to enhance health. They comprise all those individuals who provide health facilities, such as doctors, nurses, pharmacists, laboratory technicians, support workers such as finance officers, cooks, drivers, cleaners and security. Healthcare workers also include persons involved in long term care, community based care, home care and informal caregivers. *Nosocomial infections* are cross infections acquired from one patient by another or by doctors, nurses and other hospital staff while at work. The various risk factors to which healthcare professionals are exposed to are categorized as Biological, Chemical, Physical, Psychosocial, Electrical and Ergonomic. Trachoma, Leprosy, AIDS and Tetanus are some of the Surface infections to which health workers are exposed whileEmerging infectious diseases include SARS, H1N1, MERS, Chikngunya, Zika virus *etc.* A number of infectious diseases are avoidable if proper preventive measures like Hand wash (How and when), masks, sanitization, vaccination and post exposure treatments are followed by medical staff. Moreover, medical and paramedical staff with healthy habits is more likely to inculcate healthy behaviour in their patients.

**Keywords:** Acquired Immunodeficiency Syndrome (AIDS), Acute Respiratory Infections, Anaesthetic Drugs, Biohazard Level (1,2,3,4), Cleaning and Disinfectants, Cytotoxic Dugs, Droplet Infection and Nuclei, Ebola Virus Disease, External and Internal Stressor, Hepatitis Viruses C, D, E and G, HIV Infection,

* **Corresponding author Farhana Zahir:** Prism Educational Society, Aligarh, Uttar Pradesh, India; Tel: +919760986931; Email: farhanazahir@gmail.com

Leptospirosis, Middle East Respiratory Syndrome (MERS), Nosocomial Infections, Pandemic Influenza A (H1N1), Post Exposure Procedures, Structured Workplace, Surface Infections, Radiation, Zika Virus.

## INTRODUCTION

In this development oriented world, no one is exempted to the various occupational hazards originating as a result of progress. Doctors and paramedical staff spend a lifetime in keeping people healthy. According to WHO, 59 million workers are employed by healthcare sector worldwide. Ironically they are also exposed to health hazards in course of performing their duties. The risk is present during all the stages of patient care and manipulation of biological material. Unsafe working conditions and fear of infections lead to worker attrition, 57 countries have reported shortage of trained healthcare staff as reported in world health report, 2006. In order to deliver quality health care to the community and experience medicine as a rewarding career, professionals in healthcare sector also need to be healthy. Furthermore, it has been proven that medical staff with healthy habits is more likely to inculcate healthy behaviour in their patients. According to International Labour Organisation (ILO)/World Health Organisation (WHO) declaration on Health services 2005, Health care workers are all persons involved in actions whose main intent is to enhance health. They comprise all those individuals who provide health facilities, such as doctors, nurses, pharmacists and laboratory technicians. Moreover, management and support workers such as finance officers, cooks, drivers, cleaners and security guards are also included amongst healthcare workers. Healthcare workers also include persons involved in long term care, community based care, home care and informal caregivers. Many scientific reports show that healthcare workers like doctors, nurses, ward boys are exposed to various infectious diseases like HIV, Hepatitis, Tuberculosis as well as non-infectious diseases like Musculoskeletal disorders, compromised Mental health and Drug abuse.

## Hospital Acquired Infections

Hospital Acquired Infections are also called *Nosocomial infections*. They are cross infections acquired from one patient by another or by doctors, nurses and other hospital staff while at work in the hospital. Patients suffering from infectious diseases are potential source of infection for healthcare providers. The various risk factors to which healthcare professionals are exposed to are categorized as biological, chemical, physical, psychosocial, electrical and ergonomic (Fig. **1**). There are varied causes of infections in healthcare workers like direct contact, droplet infection, mosquito bites or accidents (Fig. **2**). These may be cases of certain respiratory infections viral and bacterial infections, skin infections (eczema, psoriasis), and UTI (urinary tract infections).

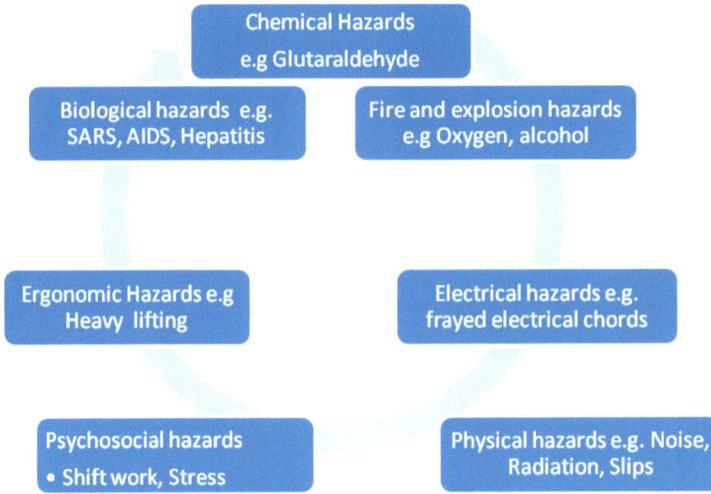

**Fig. (1).** Categories of risk factors to health care professionals.

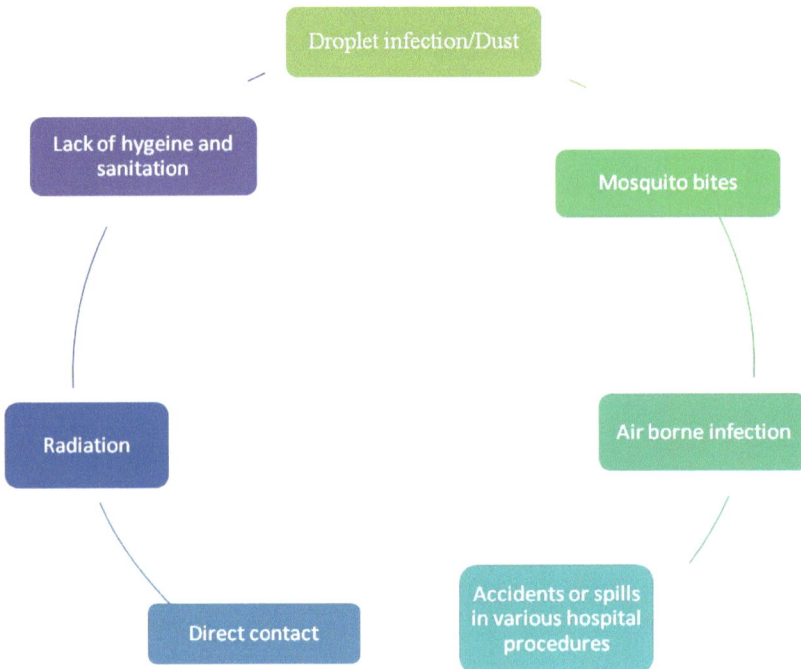

**Fig. (2).** Diverse causes of Infections in healthcare workers.

## BIOLOGICAL HAZARDS TO HEALTHCARE PROFESSIONALS

Biological hazards refer to organisms or organic matters produced by bacteria, virus, fungi, parasites and protein (Prions) that are harmful to human health. The health sector may be exposed to these agents as a result of close contact with the patients or related products like contaminated water, soil, food. The harmful effects posed to human health by biological hazards include - infections, allergy and poisoning. In general, there are four major routes of entry of microorganisms into our body (Fig. **3**).

Major Routes of Entry of infectious microbes maybe blood borne, droplet infection, contact transmission or other routes like through insect vectors or by tattooing needles. There could be one or multiple modes of entry of infectious agent into the human system. For example, the mode of transmission of Leprosy could be droplet or contact transmission. Similarly, AIDS is transmitted by sexual activity, contaminated blood transfusion, mother to child transmission (Perinatal) through placenta during delivery or by breast feeding.

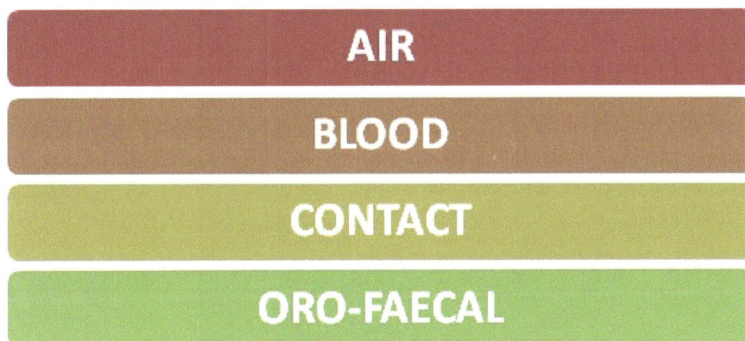

**AIR**

**BLOOD**

**CONTACT**

**ORO-FAECAL**

**Fig. (3).** Major of routes of entry of micro organisms/pathogens.

### Types of Air Borne Infections

1. **Droplet infection:** Droplet nuclei are dried residues of droplets, 1-10 μm which are formed by coughing, sneezing or aerosols. The droplet nuclei may retain virulence for a long time. 1-5 μm droplets are easily drawn to lungs alveoli and maybe retained, leading to a number of diseases like tuberculosis, influenza, chickenpox *etc.*

2. **Dust:** Large droplets generated during coughing, talking, sneezing settle down on the floor, furniture, bedding, clothes, linen and other objects in the immediate vicinity becoming part of the dust. During sweeping, dusting and bedmaking the dust is released into air and becomes once again airborne.

## Surface Infections Seen in Health Care Providers

Trachoma, Leprosy, AIDS and Tetanus are some of the surface infections to which health workers are exposed (Fig. **4**).

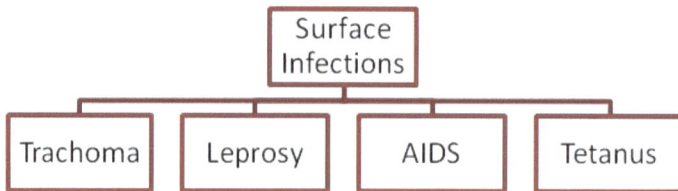

**Fig. (4).**  Surface infections seen in healthcare workers.

## *Acquired Immunodeficiency Syndrome (AIDS)*

There is a small, but definite occupational risk of HIV transmission to health care and laboratory personnel who work with HIV containing materials and sharps. According to an estimate 600,000 to 800,000 workers are stuck with needles and sharps each year in the hospital environment. Hospital air, dust, linen, bed clothes, furniture, sink, basins, doors and door handles all become source of infection for hospital staff including doctors, nurses, lab boys multi task staff (MTS). The hospital staff which comes in close contact with the patient is more prone to get infection (Fig. **5**).

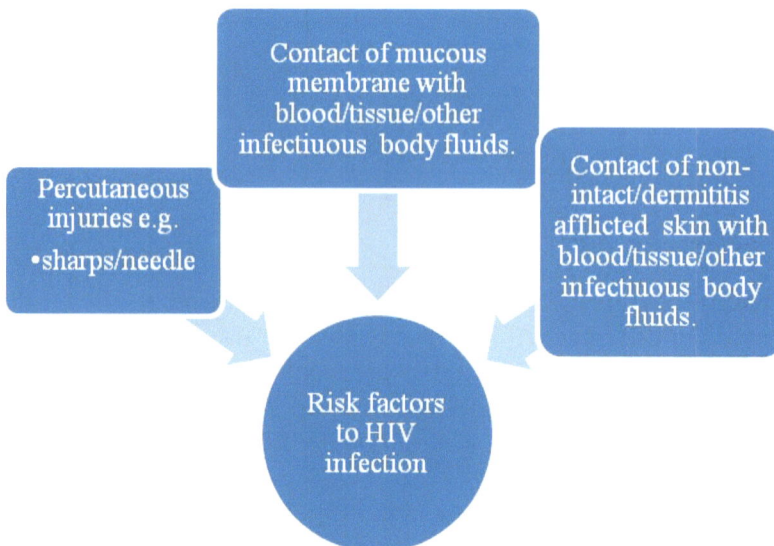

**Fig. (5).**  Contributing factors to HIV infection in healthcare workers.

Trachoma is a chronic infectious disease of the eye caused by *Chlamydia trachomatis.* It is transmitted eye to eye by direct or indirect contact with fomites or infected ocular discharge.

Leprosy or Hansen disease is a chronic infectious disease induced by *Mycobacterium leprae.* The mode of transmission of leprosy could be through droplet or contact transmission. Tetanus is an acute disease caused by the exotoxin of *Clostridium tetani.* Its infection is transmitted by contamination of wounds with tetanus spores (Fig. **6**).

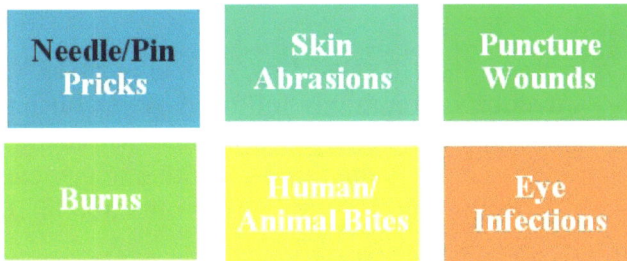

| Needle/Pin Pricks | Skin Abrasions | Puncture Wounds |
| Burns | Human/ Animal Bites | Eye Infections |

**Fig. (6).** Contributing factors to HIV infection in healthcare workers.

## Respiratory Infections Seen in Health Care Providers

Commonly seen infections like chicken pox, small pox, Measles, Mumps, Rubella *etc* in healthcare workers are listed (Table **1**) along with their causative agent and

**Table 1.** List of some common Respiratory Infections seen in healthcare providers.

| Disease | Causative Agent and Mode of Transmission |
|---|---|
| Small pox | Variola virus, droplet infection and droplet nuclei |
| Chicken pox | Varicella -zoster, droplet infection and droplet nuclei (aerosol) |
| Measles | Myxovirus,droplet infection and droplet nuclei |
| Rubella | Togavirus, droplets from nose and throat and droplet nuclei. |
| Mumps | Myxovirus,droplet infection |
| Influenza | Influenza virus, droplet infection and droplet nuclei |
| Tuberclulosis | *Mycobacterium tuberculosis,*Droplet infection and droplet nuclei |
| Pandemic Influenza A ($H_1N_1$) | Pandemic Influenza A ($H_1N_1$) 2009 virus, droplet nuclei |
| Meningococcal Meningits | Neissaria Meningitis, droplet infection |
| Acute Respiratory infections | Bacteria and Virus, droplet nuclei |
| SARS (Severe Acute respiratory syndrome) | Corona virus, respiratory droplet or fomites |

mode of transmission. The respiratory infections are mostly transmitted from person to person by droplet infection and by droplet nuclei. Most of the healthcare workers are infected by "face to face" (Personal contact). Respiratory tract is the common portal of infection.

### Small Pox

It is an acute infectious disease caused by Variola virus. World has been declared small pox free in 1980 by World Health Organisation.

### Chicken Pox

It is an acute highly infectious disease caused by Varicella–zoster virus (Human Herpes virus). Primary infection is commonly followed by establishment of latent infection in the sensory ganglion of the cranial nerves and also in the spinal dorsal root ganglia. Reduction in the cell mediated immunity due to any cause may lead to reactivation of the virus resulting in Herpes –zoster infection in 10-30% of the cases.

### Measles

It is an acute highly infectious disease seen in mostly young adults caused by Myxoviruses. Measles infection is prevented by MMR vaccine. The disease is currently on rise particularly in health care workers who are frequent international travellers. Measles during pregnancy is associated with spontaneous abortion and premature delivery. Mild to severe measles is seen in infants born to infected mothers, therefore, these infants should be immunized immediately to prevent infection. According to WHO during 2000-2014 measles vaccination prevented mortality of 17.1 million.

### Rubella or German Measles

It is an acute childhood and young adults'infection. Infection in early pregnancy may result in  serious congenital defects including  death of the fetus, this is known as **Congenital Rubella Syndrome (CRS)**. According to WHO-CRS rate is highest in African and South-East Asia due to low rates of vaccination. Rubella infection is prevented by **MMR** vaccine.

### Mumps

It is an acute infectious disease caused by RNA virus of the family para-myxoviradiae. Infection in early trimester may result in spontaneous abortion. The disease is currently on rise particularly in health care workers who are frequent international travellers. Mumps infection is prevented by MMR vaccine.

## *Influenza*

It is an acute respiratory tract infection caused by influenza virus. WHO issues guidelines every year to contain H and N components of the virus in the vaccine as the vaccine has limited success so far. Seasonal Influenza vaccination is recommended by more than 40 countries including US particularly for healthcare workers. Influenza infection during pregnancy is associated with spontaneous abortion and premature delivery.

## *Tuberculosis (TB)*

It is a public health problem worldwide. *Mycobacterium tuberculosis* causes tuberculosis. The disease usually affects lungs but extra pulmonary tuberculosis is also common. The disease is transmitted from a person with infectious pulmonary tuberculosis to others by droplet nuclei which are aerosolised by coughing, sneezing or speaking. Several studies have clearly demonstrated that TB patients whose sputum contains AFB (Acid Fast Bacilli) Visible by microscopy are the most likely to transmit the infection. Patients with sputum smear negative/culture positive are less infectious. Patients with culture negative pulmonary disease and extra pulmonary tuberculosis are non-infectious. Crowding in poorly ventilated rooms with patients is also a contributing factor towards disease. The patients with infectious TB should be placed in negative pressure room with 6 or more air changes per hour.

The probability of contact with a person who has an infectious form of TB and the duration of exposure and the degree of infectiousness of the case increases the likelihood of transmission. It is a major cause of death worldwide. Due to above contributing factors health care professionals interacting with patients are more susceptible to the bacillus infection. The healthcare workers should wear N95 mask. The World Health Organization declared TB a "**global health emergency**" in 1993 and in 2006, the Stop TB partnership developed a Global Plan to Stop TB that aims to save 14 million between its launch and 2015.The multitasking staff in third world countries like Bangladesh is unaware of the causative agents and preventive measures of the disease, hence such staff must be imparted with adequate knowledge regarding causation, transmission and prevention of the disease [1]. Smoking aggravates the risk of the disease and high hygiene standards decrease the incidence of the disease.

## *Pandemic Influenza A ($H_1N_1$)*

It is discussed under emerging infectious diseases.

## *Meningitis*

It is an acute infectious disease caused by *Nisseria meningitides*, a gram negative bacteria. The port of entry is nasopharynx and the disease is spread mainly by droplet infection. The disease is fatal in 5-10% of cases and 15-20% of survivors suffer from permanent neurological damage. Close contact with patients increases the chances of Meningococcal illness in healthcare workers. Currently polysaccharide, polysaccharide-protein conjugate vaccine is available against the infection. Smoking aggravates the risk of the disease [2].

## *Acute Respiratory infections*

Acute Respiratory infections result in inflammation of the respiratory tract. They are referred as **Acute Respiratory Infections** (ARI) of upper or lower respiratory tract depending on the site of the infection. They become significant cause of morbidity and mortality. The pathogens that result in ARI (Fig. **7**) are numerous bacteria (like, *Haemophilus influenzae, klebsiella pneumoniae, Legionella pneumo- phila, Staphylococcus pyogenes, Streptococcus pneumonia, Streptococcus pyogenes)* and viruses (Adeno virus, Entero virus, influenza virus, Rhino virus, Corona virus). Healthcare workers are exposed to these air borne infections as they are involved in care and handling of the sick. Improving hygiene at workplace may result in decreased incidence of Acute Respiratory Infections.

## *SARS (Severe Acute Respiratory Syndrome)*

It is discussed under emerging infectious diseases.

### Bacteria

• *Haemophilus influenzae, Klebsiella pneumoniae, Legionella pneumophila, Staphylococcus pyogenes, Streptococcus pneumonia, Streptococcus pyogenes*

### Viruses

• Adeno virus, Entero virus, Influenza virus, Rhino virus, Corona virus

**Fig. (7).** Pathogens causing acute respiratory diseases.

## Intestinal Infections

Intestinal Infections seen in health care providers are summarized in Table **2**.

**Table 2. List of some common Intestinal Infections seen in health care providers.**

| DISEASE | • CAUSATIVE AGENT AND MODE OF TRANSMISSION |
|---|---|
| Hepatitis A | • Hepatitis A virus, predominantly faecal-oral transmission, rarely parenteral or sexual transmission. |
| Hepatitis B | • Hepatitis B Virus predominantly parenteral rarely sexual transmission or perinatal transmission. |
| Hepatitis C | • Hepatitis C Virus, predominantly parenteral rarely sexual transmission or perinatal transmission. |
| Hepatitis D | • Hepatitis D Virus, predominantly parenteral |
| Hepatitis E | • Hepatitis E Virus, predominantly faecal-oral transmission. |
| Hepatitis G | • Hepatitis G Virus, trnsfusion through blood transfusion. |
| Acute diarroheal diseases | • Bacteria, Virus or protozoa, predominantly faecal-oral transmission. |
| Cholera | • *Vibrio cholerae*, faecal oral and direct contact. |
| Thyphoid | • *Salmonella typhi,* faecal oral and direct contact. |
| Amoebiasis | • *Entamoeba histolytica,* faecal oral and direct contact. |

## *Viral Hepatitis*

It is characterised by the infection of the liver caused by viruses. Percutaneous exposure is a known event in health care facilities. Many pathogens are acquired through this type of exposure. Today in addition to HAV and HBV, Hepatitis viruses C, D, E and G are also known etiological agents of viral hepatitis.

### Hepatitis A Virus

Infectious hepatitis / epidemic jaundice is mainly caused by Hepatitis A virus. It is transmitted *via* faecal-oral route, very rarely it may be transmitted by parenteral route or by skin penetration during the stage of viraemia.

### Hepatitis B Virus

Serum hepatitis is mainly caused by Hepatitis B virus. It is transmitted by parenteral route by sharps/needle injury or through handling of infected blood. The carrier rate of HbsAg in hospital staff has been found to be higher than general population. Certain subgroups like nurses and laboratory personnel are at high risk particularly operating room staff. Serological screening and vaccination of high risk group is highly recommended.

### Hepatitis C Virus

It is mainly transmitted by infectious blood, sex or sharing of personal items by an infected person.

### Hepatitis D Virus

It is mainly transmitted by contaminated blood parenterally.

### Hepatitis E Virus (Non-A Non-B also known as HNANB)

It is mainly transmitted through contaminated water or food by indirect contamination by faecal matter carrying the virus.

### Hepatitis G

This virus is associated by blood transfusion.

### Diarrhoea

It is the passage of loose liquid watery stools usually more than three times a day. A flowchart indicating various categories of causative agents; virus, bacteria and fungi of diarrhoeal diseases in healthcare sector is shown Fig. (**8**). Faecal-oral transmission may be water-borne, food-borne or direct *via* fingers, fomites or dirt.

### Cholera

Itis an acute diarrhoeal disease caused by comma shaped bacterium *Vibrio cholera*. Adequate environmental management is necessary to contain the disease in healthcare personnel. The disease is global threat to healthcare staff particularly in developing countries due to lack of basic hygiene procedures as the transmi-

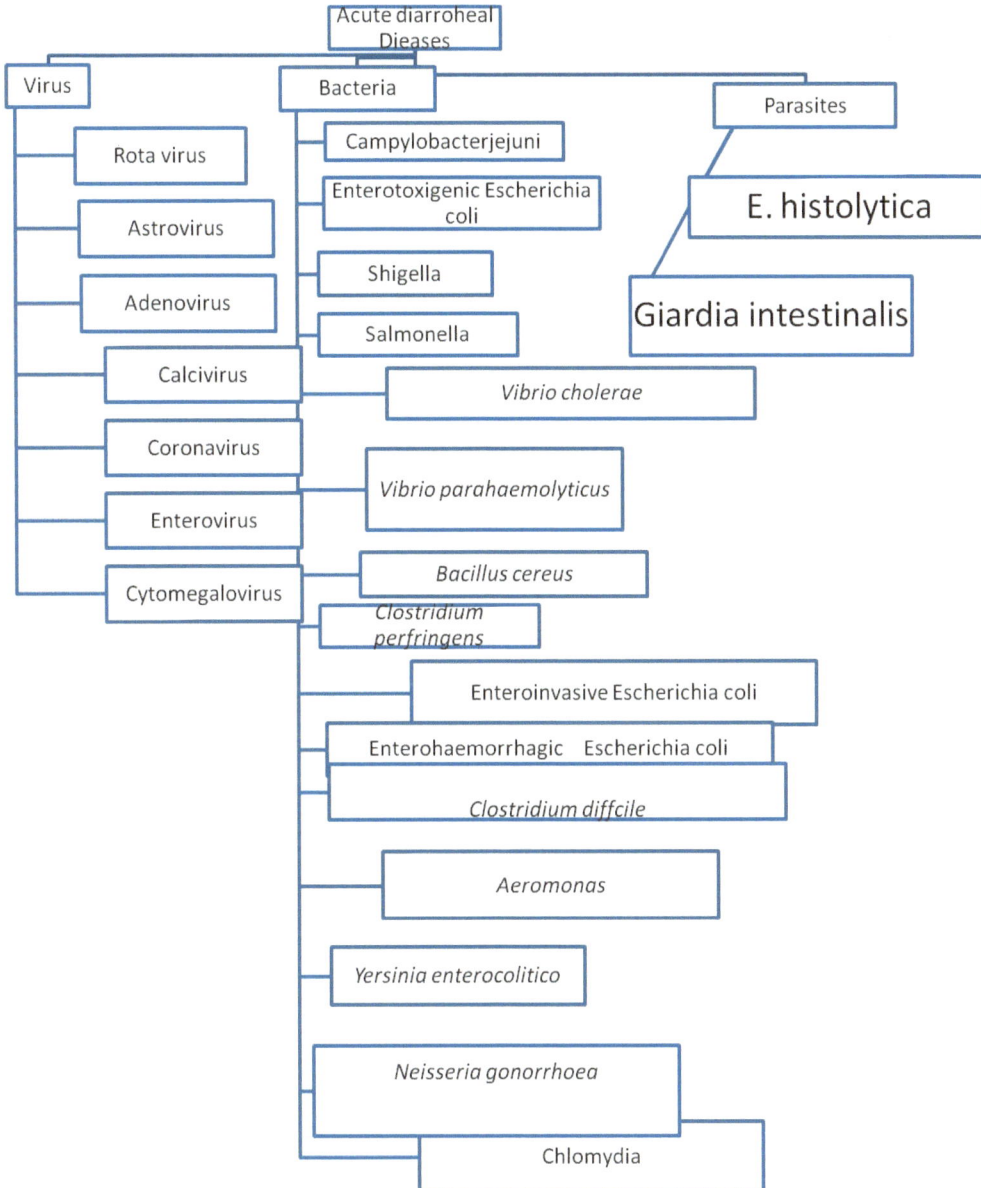

**Fig. (8).** Flowchart showing various causative agents for acute diarrhoeal diseases in healthcare sector.

ssion occurs from man to man *via* direct contact through contaminated fingers while carelessly handling excreta vomit of patients, contaminated linen and fomites.

## *Typhoid*

It is fever caused by *S. typhi*. The primary source of infection is faeces and urine of cases or carriers. The secondary sources are contaminated water, food, finger and flies. Popularisation of health education/sanitation/personal hygiene to hospital staff will minimise the risk of disease.

## *Amoebiasis*

It is caused by *E. Histolytica*. The mode of transmission of amoebiasis is faeco-oral and sexual. Vectors (like cockroaches, rodents, flies) carry cyst and contaminate food and drinks. Strict hygiene and following sanitation rules can reduce risk of disease in general and healthcare staff.

## Zoonotic Infections in Healthcare Sector

Zoonotic diseases are infections the agents of which are naturally transmitted between vertebrate animals and men (Fig. **9**). Antropozoonosis include infections that are transmitted to men from lower vertebrate animals.

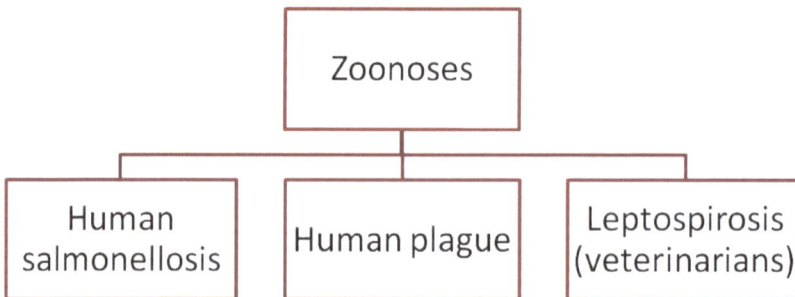

**Fig. (9).** Diagram showing common zoonotic infections in healthcare sector.

## *Human Salmonellosis*

In healthcare workers Salmonellosis is spread due to eating raw eggs and undercooked meat in hospital kitchens [3].

## *Human Plague*

It is caused by *Y. Pestis*, and transmitted to men by infected flea bites, occa-sionally by direct contact with the tissue of infected animals or droplet infection from cases of Pneumonic plague. Beside other measures, disinfection of sputum discharges and articles soiled by the patient should be carried out. Aseptic precautions should be taken while handling the dead bodies. Mass destruction of fleas and rodents by application of effective insecticide should also be carried out.

## *Leptospirosis*

It is animal infection by leptospira (Spirochaetes). Human infections are due to occupational exposure to the urine of infected animals in veterinarians. Control measures include preventing exposure to potentially contaminated water, reducing contamination by rodent control. Proper disposal of waste and health education is also helpful.

## Arthropod Borne Infections in Healthcare Sector

Anopheles, Aedes and Culex mosquitoes are vector mosquitoes prevalent in developing countries of Asia, Africa, Oceania, South and Central America. Japanese Encephalitis [4], Yellow fever, malaria, West Nile Virus and Dengue fever are diseases caused by mosquito bite. Establishment of hospitals in remote areas expose healthcare staff to these arthropod infections (Fig. **10**). Vector control and personal protection is successful to contain such infections.

## Emerging Infectious Diseases in Healthcare Sector

They are a group of diseases whose incidence in humans has increased in the past two decades or threaten to increase in near future. The hospital and related staff is particularly a high risk cohort for such disorders (Fig. **11**).

## *Zika Virus*

It is transmitted by *Aedes agypti*. Clearing rodents will decrease the chance of infection. It is currently an epidemic in Latin America and Caribbean. The Offsprings of healthcare workers suffer from microcephaly, therefore information regarding prevention of infection must be spread among staff of child bearing age.

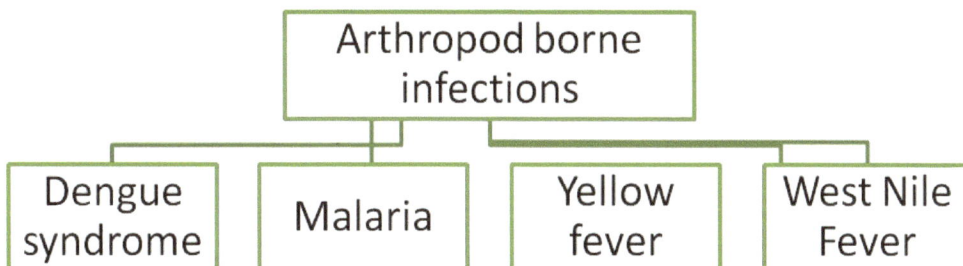

**Fig. (10).** Diagram showing common arthropod borne infections in healthcare sector.

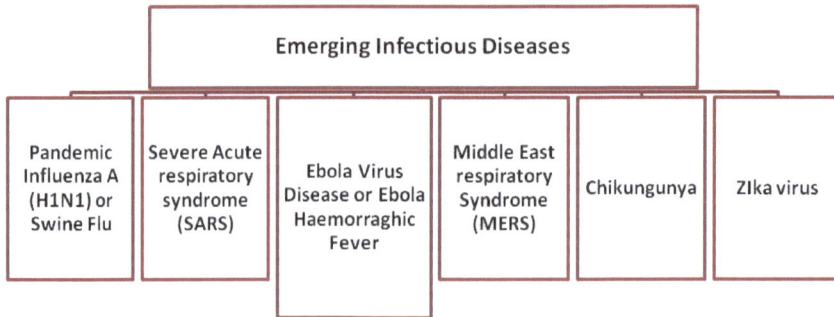

**Fig. (11).** Emerging infectious diseases in healthcare sector.

## *Ebola Virus Disease or Ebola Haemorraghic Fever*

It is a highly contagious viral fever erupted in Africa in December 2013. Healthcare givers must follow safe practices like proper hand wash. Relapse of infection in CNS is observed, therefore severe vigilance is required to save patient and break the new transmission chain.

## *Pandemic Influenza A (H1N1)*

In 2011, Influenza A was given a new nomenclature H1N1. H1N1 commonly known as **Swine Flu** was declared **pandemic** in the year 2009. H1N1virus can infect the lower respiratory tract leading to progressive pneumonia especially in children, pregnant women and young adults. H1N1 infection during pregnancy is associated with spontaneous abortion and premature delivery. Due to high risk of secondary infection and limited treatment options WHO recommends all healthcare workers to be immunised against the disease. Since, the vaccine reduces the risk of the disease but is not 100% effective public education regarding preventive measures is essential. Powered **Air Purifying Respirators** are now recommended by board of Health Sciences Policy, Institute of Medicine, USA for prevention of **H1N1 and Ebola virus** infection. European countries usually recommend leave to infected workers to prevent spread of infection.

## Severe Acute Respiratory Syndrome (SARS)

It is spread by a corona virus. It was first reported in China.

It is a common viral infection caused by a new strain of corona virus. SARS outbreak in 2003 led to conclusion that preventive measures are key players to contain the epidemic. SARS protocol should be strictly followed at workplace. The procedures generating aerosol like endotracheal intubation, mechanical ventilation, bronchoscopy, nebulisation may increase the transmission of the

SARS virus. Health care workers involved in these procedures are more prone to get SARS and account for 21% of all the cases.

## Middle East Respiratory Syndrome

The deadly infection was first reported to spread in 2012, by CoronaVirus in Gulf region through animal reservoir dromedary camels. It has been reported in 26 countries including Korea. Currently there is no treatment or vaccination for MERS. Therefore, strict isolation of patient is advised to avoid triggering epidemic. The healthcare staff is vulnerable to infection if they ignore warnings. Smoking or previous infection aggravate the disease.

## Chikungunya

It is caused by chikungunya virus belonging to the genus Alphavirus, carried through mosquito bite. There is long lasting impact of chikungunya on limb extremities particularly those having history of Rheumatologic disease. Currently there is no vaccine or effective drug against the infection, therefore vector prevention is necessary.

## Biohazard Levels

A material which poses threat to cells or tissue is called biohazard. Hazardous biological substances are classified according to the intensity of threat into four **Biohazard Levels** (Fig. **12**). The level of required biological safety measures (BSL) enhances as the level of biohazard increases (Fig. **13**).

## Biohazard Levels 1

This includes non-pathogenic and non-infectious, bacteria. They require **Biosafety level 1** like basic laboratory gloves and masks ay they fall under least risk group.

**Example:** *Escherichia coli*

## Biohazard Levels 2

This includes mild disease causing bacteria and viruses. They require **Biosafety**

**level 2** additional safety measures like autoclaving is used in addition to standard laboratory measures for biosafety level 1.

**Example:** *Staphylococcs aureus*

| Biohazard Level 1 | Biohazard Level 2 | Biohazard Level 3 | Biohazard Level 4 |
|---|---|---|---|
| Non-infectious Bacteria and viruses | Infectious biological agents which cause mild disease, treatment is available. | Infectious biological agents which cause severe disease, treatment is available, No vaccine. | Infectious agents that can cause severe to fatal disease in humans for which no vaccines or other treatments exist. |

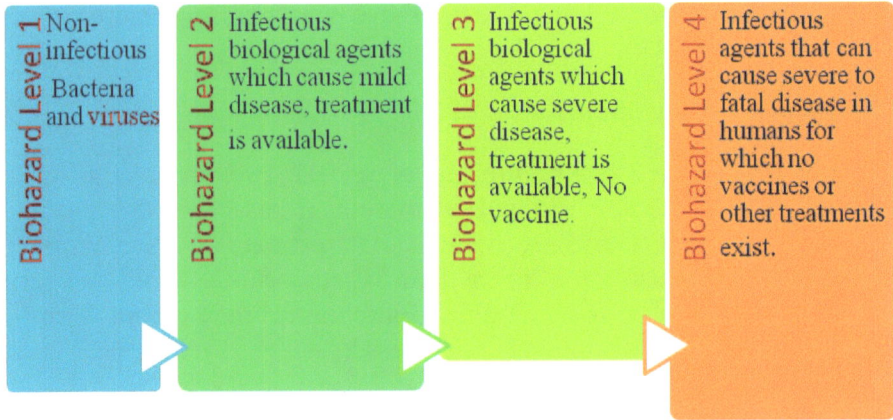

**Fig. (12).** Biohazard levels are classified according to the intensity of infection.

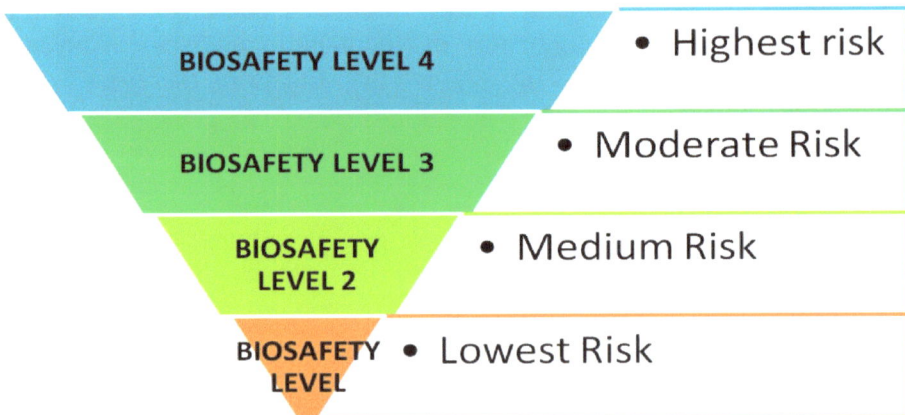

**BIOSAFETY LEVEL 4** • Highest risk

**BIOSAFETY LEVEL 3** • Moderate Risk

**BIOSAFETY LEVEL 2** • Medium Risk

**BIOSAFETY LEVEL** • Lowest Risk

**Fig. (13).** Biohazard levels are classified according to the intensity of infection.

## Biohazard Levels 3

This includes agents causing severe to fatal infections but treatments are available and vaccines may exist. They require **Biosafety level 3** safety measures like controlled access to hospitals/laboratory, respirators and immunization (if available) for workers in addition to standard laboratory measures for biosafety level 2.

**Example:** *Mycobacterium tuberculosis*.

## Biohazard Levels 4

This includes bacteria and viruses causing dangerous and fatal infections, no treatments and vaccines exist for this category. They generate fatal aerosols. They require **Biosafety level 4** safety measures like isolated zones, structured buildings, special suits in addition to standard laboratory measures for biosafety level 3. This is highest risk category.

**Example:** Zika virus

## CHEMICAL HAZARDS OR PHARMACEUTICAL EXPOSURE TO MEDICAL AND PARAMEDICAL STAFF

In health sector chemical risks are due to harmful chemicals/pharmaceuticals/toxic dusts used (Table **3**). Some chemicals may cause respiratory illnesses, skin allergies. They may also have harmful effect on blood and other organs of the body.

**Table 3. Various classes of chemicals attributing towards health hazards in Health Professionals.**

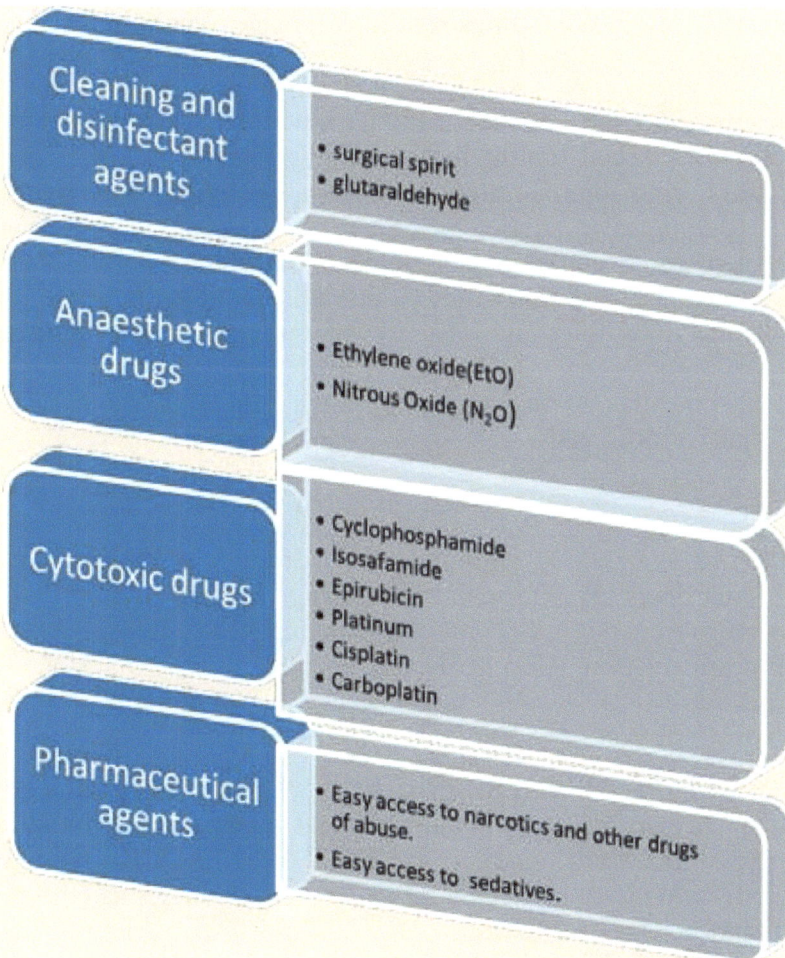

| Cleaning and disinfectant agents | • surgical spirit<br>• glutaraldehyde |
| Anaesthetic drugs | • Ethylene oxide(EtO)<br>• Nitrous Oxide (N$_2$O) |
| Cytotoxic drugs | • Cyclophosphamide<br>• Isosafamide<br>• Epirubicin<br>• Platinum<br>• Cisplatin<br>• Carboplatin |
| Pharmaceutical agents | • Easy access to narcotics and other drugs of abuse.<br>• Easy access to sedatives. |

Workers may be exposed to hazardous pharmaceutical compounds from manufacture, transit, distribution, use and disposal. The workers in the pharmaceutical manufacturing sector, distributors, pharmacists, nursing staff, operation theatre staff, physicians and persons working in research laboratories all include populations under high risk of exposure to unwanted drugs. The adverse effects of pharmaceutical exposure maybe broadly divided into acute and chronic effects.

Acute effects include skin rashes.

Chronic effects include reproductive health problems and cancers.

## Conditions for Exposure to Hazardous Drugs (Clinical and Non-Clinical Staff)

The main routes of exposure are through inhalation, skin contact, accidental ingestion or injection. Various activities resulting in exposure of clinical and non-clinical workers are:

◉Surgical procedures like intra-operative and intra-peritoneal chemotherapy.
◉Generating dust while reconstituting lyophilizedor powdered drugs.
◉Creating aerosol during administration of drugs either by direct IV route or IV infusion while expelling air.
  ○ Contact while cleaning spills or counting uncoated tablets.
  ○ Contact with contaminated body fluids, dressing, clothing, linen *etc.*
  ○ Disposal of hazardous drugs and waste like partially filled vials, undispensed

    products, used needles, syringes, gloves, gowns, underpads and containers such as IV bags or drug vials.

### *Mutagenicity*

Pharmacists and nurses handling anti- neoplastic drugs at workplace are more prone to genotoxic effects [5]. Chromosomal damage leading to micronucleated lymphocytes is more frequent in hospital workers exposed to ionising radiations than in controls despite very low levels of exposure [6].

### *Cancer*

Healthcare workers exposed to anti-neoplastic drugs have been found to be more susceptible to cancer particularly leukemia [7] and breast cancer. Incidence of lung, thyroid, breast and uterus cancer were found to be increased while cervix and liver cancer was found to be decreased in Taiwanese nurses as compared to general population [8].

### *Reproductive Health Problems*

Adverse reproductive events include increased fetal loss (spontaneous abortions), low birth weight, infertility, congenital effects depending on the duration of exposure to anaesthetic gases (like nitrous oxide), anti-neoplastic drugs or biologic agents (like HIV, Cytomegala, Varicella and Rubella) or ionizing radiations.

### *Occupational Asthma and Allergies*

Work related agents like animal proteins, enzymes, natural rubber, latex, reactive chemicals *e.g.* glutarladehyde and cleansing products encountered by health care workers can also cause allergic problems such as asthma.

Exposure to latex may result in allergic reactions in health care personnel and others who frequently wear latex gloves. Allergic reaction to Latex may be serious and can very rarely be fatal.

## PSYCHOSOCIAL RISKS TO HEALTHCARE PROFESSIONALS

The likelihood of lifestyle disorders *e.g.*, hypertension, diabetes, cardiovascular diseases *etc.* is lower amongst medicos, though there is evidence of high rate of mental problems, alcoholism and drug abuse among certain subgroups of doctors (Fig. **14**). There are multiple internal and external stressors in medicine. Personality traits like dedication, commitment, sense of responsibility, competitiveness and altruism are **internal stressors** which contribute to compromised mental state. Depression and anxiety owing to **external stressors'** like shift work, extra-long working hours coupled with fierce competition within the profession contribute to high suicide rate among the doctors. Recently violence against healthcare staff particularly physicians has emerged as one of the biggest psychosocial problems.

## ERGONOMIC RISKS TO HEALTHCARE PROFESSIONALS

A number of healthcare providers are affected by MSD (Musculoskeletal Disorders). In case of medicos such disorders result due to patient handling, working in odd time schedule, adverse working environment, prolonged sitting/standing, awkward and repetitive working postures as in operation theatres and during routine nursing work. The lumber region is most affected (63.1%) due to work in nurses followed by cervical region, shoulders, wrist and hand [9].

## ELECTRICAL RISKS TO HEALTHCARE PROFESSIONALS

A lot of electronic equipment is used now- a- days by healthcare staff. Short circuits, frayed cords or a defective gadget might cause accident or in extreme cases fire causing distress to healthcare staff.

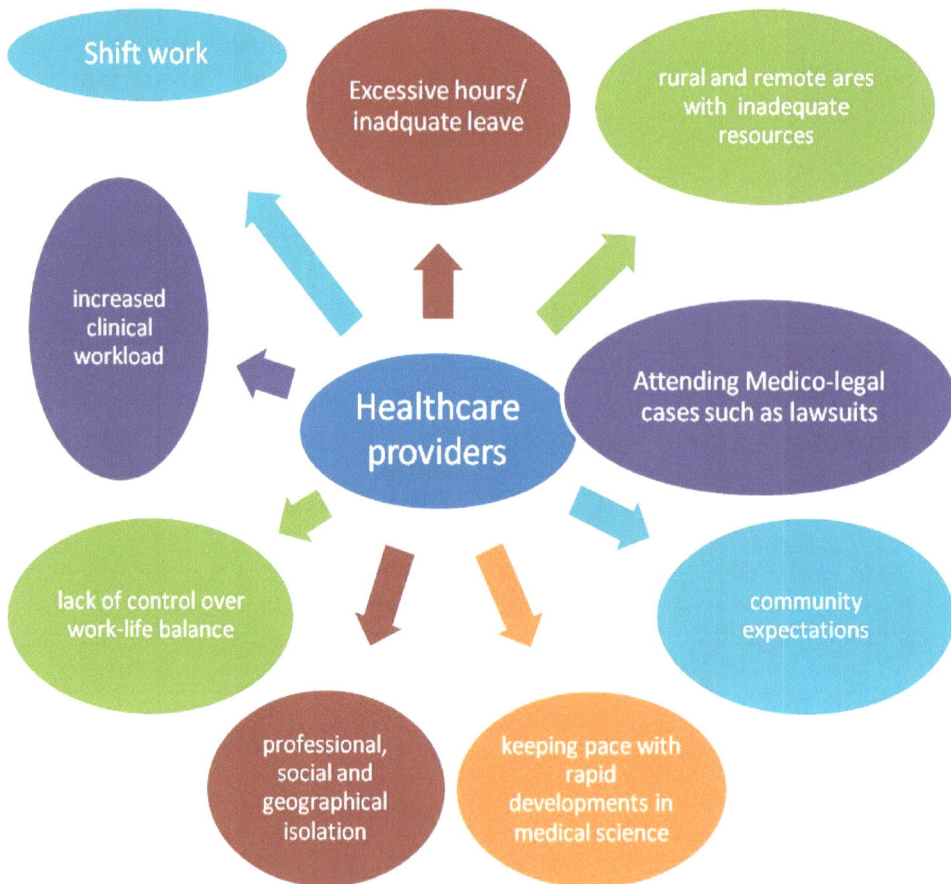

**Fig. (14).** Factors associated with psychosocial risk to healthcare professionals.

## PHYSICAL HAZARDS TO HEALTHCARE PROFESSIONALS
### Physical Hazards

Environment which may have adverse effect on health are extremes of temperature, light, noise, vibrations, radiation.

### Radiation Hazards

Ionizing radiations are used in many modern diagnostic and surgical procedures. They comprise largest man made source of medical radiation to the medical and paramedical staff. X- rays, Computed Tomography (CT), nuclear medicine procedures and interventional radiology are some of the prime sources of exposure. Interventional radiologists receive non uniform radiational, occupational doses through-out their working time. A twenty-year study on US radiologists found them to be more susceptible to diseases of eye including cataract [10].

For example, cardiologists and supportive staff working in cardiology suite is prone to occupational radiation exposure particularly to the lens of their eyes while performing percutaneous coronary intervention electrophysiology procedures, diagnostic invasive coronary angiogram and other interventional cardiology procedures [11]. Endoscopists performing endoscopic procedures *e.g.* Endoscopic Retrograde Cholangiopancreatography (ERCP) are also exposed to radiations [12].

## PREVENTIVE MEASURES FOR PREVENTION OF INFECTIONS TO HEALTHCARE PROFESSIONALS

There is no foolproof barrier for prevention of diseases as the rate of exposure of infections to healthcare professionals is very high. Simple personal protective equipment (Figs. **15** and **16**) and simple daily hygiene practices (Fig. **17**) and antisepsis go a long way in bringing down the rate of diseases. Emergency medical workers play an important role in providing pre-hospital medical care.Though the infections in hospitals can be controlled by keeping strict quality control, the emergency medical personnel are constantly exposed to infections. Assessment of risk for emergency medical staff or para medical staff is difficult and expectedly quite high.Their immune system is also compromised as a result of working under pressure.

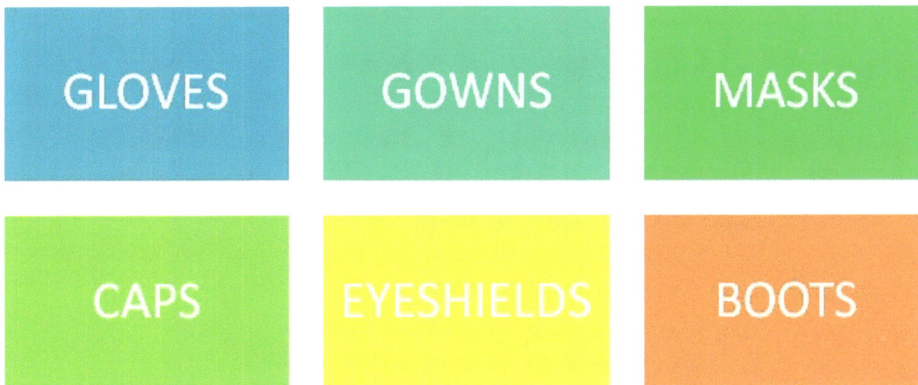

| | | |
|---|---|---|
| GLOVES | GOWNS | MASKS |
| CAPS | EYESHIELDS | BOOTS |

**Fig. (15).** Use of Personal Protective Equipment is necessary.

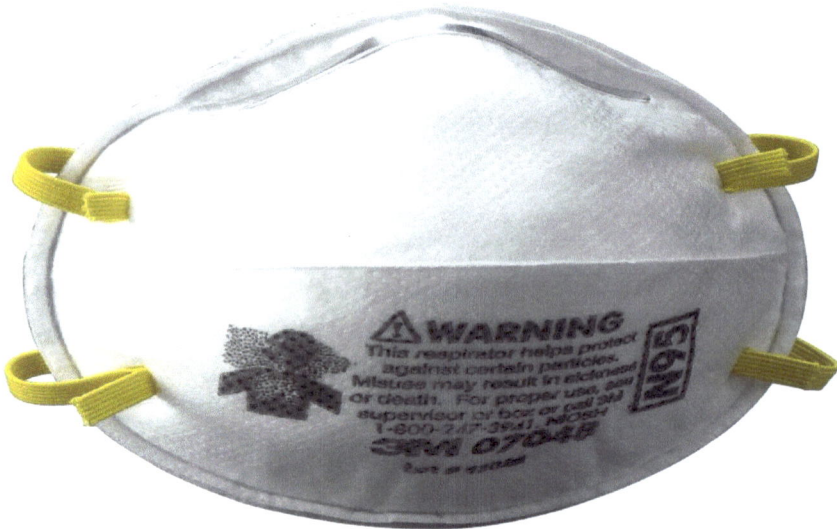

**Fig. (16).**  N 95 MASK is better than simple mask.

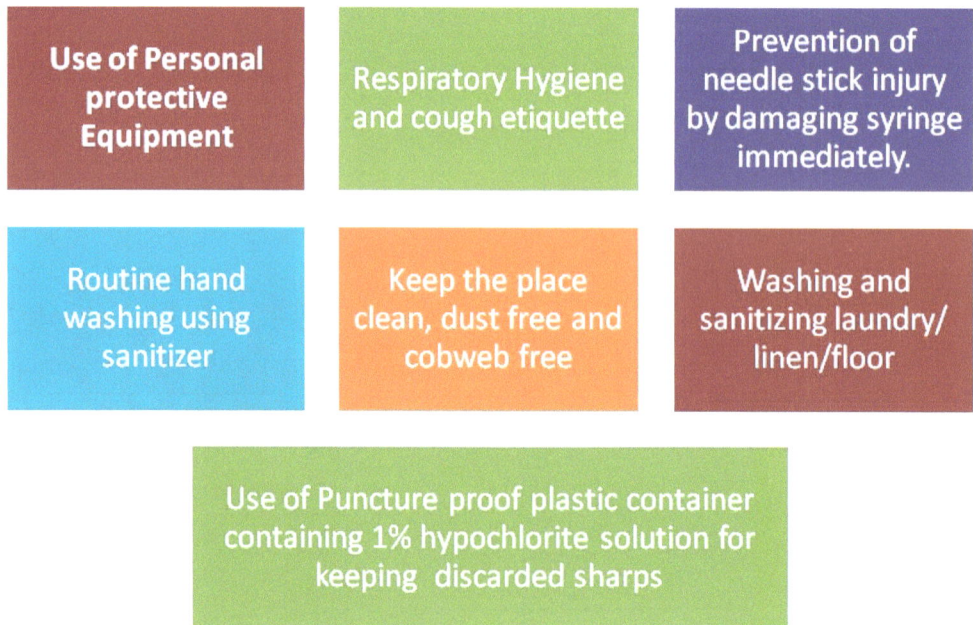

| | | |
|---|---|---|
| **Use of Personal protective Equipment** | Respiratory Hygiene and cough etiquette | Prevention of needle stick injury by damaging syringe immediately. |
| Routine hand washing using sanitizer | Keep the place clean, dust free and cobweb free | Washing and sanitizing laundry/ linen/floor |

Use of Puncture proof plastic container containing 1% hypochlorite solution for keeping  discarded sharps

**Fig. (17).**  Summary of Simple Practices for prevention of diseases.

## PREVENTIVE MEASURES

### Hand Washing and Antisepsis

a. Before and after touching a patient for examination or applying gel, giving face mask.
b. Before and after any aseptic procedure like lumber puncture/ surgical procedure.
c. After body fluid exposure risk like wound dressing/skin lesion care/ drawing and manipulating any fluid sample, soiled material, urinal, bedpan, medical instruments *etc.*
d. After touching patient surroundings like bed, side table, monitoring alarm *etc.*

Needle stick injuries are well recognised all over the world. These injuries can be minimized by use of puncture proof plastic container containing 1% hypochlorite solution for keeping discarded sharps.

• Needle damage using needle destroyer after every use.

### *Vaccinations*

Ideally all medical personnel should be vaccinated with **Hepatitis B** vaccine before they begin their career. The dose for adults is 10-20 micrograms initially and the dose should be repeated again at 1 and 6 months (0,1,6). Deltoid muscle is preferred for injection as injection in the gluteal region often results in deposition of vaccine in fat rather than muscle, with serologic conversion. **The vaccine against HBV also protects from liver cancer.**

Two types of HAV are used worldwide inactivated and live attenuated. The complete vaccination schedule consists of two doses into the deltoid muscle.

Two types of oral cholera vaccines are available. Typhoid vaccines are also available.

### Preventive Medicine

A recent meta- analysis report suggests that 6-12 months of preventive TB therapy using isoniazid resulted in a lower incidence of active tuberculosis as compared with individuals with positive tuberculin test [13].

### Post Exposure Procedures

For HIV infections a four-week basic regimen of Zidovudine and lamivudine, Lamivudine and Stavudine or Didanosine and Stavudine should be taken [14].

## Simple Practices for Prevention of Diseases

1. Powered Air Purifying Respirators are now recommended by board of Health Sciences Policy, Institute of Medicine, USA for prevention of H1N1 and Ebola virus infection. European countries usually recommend leave to infected workers to prevent spread of infection.
2. Mobile phones are infected by various pathogens. They should be disinfected regularly.
3. SARS protocol should be strictly followed at workplace.
4. A **structured workplace** helps healthcare staff to work in case of biological disaster like SARS or H1N1.
5. Public education regarding diseases helps to remove or diminish stigma associated with the disease in the family of health care worker, this in turn will lead to stress free health caregivers.
6. Media coverage regarding a disease should be monitored to stay sensible, otherwise the morale of healthcare worker is compromised.
7. Multi tasking staff and healthcare workers should be empowered.
8. Aseptic precautions should be taken while handling the dead bodies. Mass destruction of fleas and rodents by application of effective insecticide should also be carried out to prevent diseases like plague.
9. Clearing the bushes (Fig. **18**) cleaning rodents/stray dogs prevent infections like malaria, dengue, plagues and leptospirosis.
10. Chlorinating water supplies, boiling drinking water.
11. Tutorial initiatives are effective in dissemination of information regarding disease amongst healthcare staff.

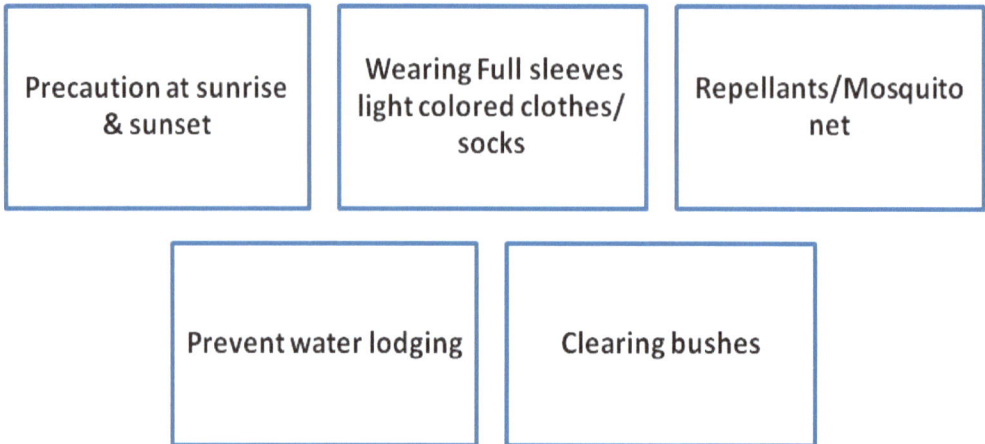

| Precaution at sunrise & sunset | Wearing Full sleeves light colored clothes/ socks | Repellants/Mosquito net |
|---|---|---|
| Prevent water lodging | Clearing bushes | |

**Fig. (18).** Routine precautions for preventing arthropod borne infections like malaria and dengue.

## CONSENT FOR PUBLICATION

Not applicable.

## CONFLICT OF INTEREST

The authors confirm that this chapter contents have no conflict of interest.

## ACKNOWLEDGEMENTS

Declared none.

## REFERENCES

[1]     Islam QS, Islam MA, Islam S, Ahmed SM. Prevention and control of tuberculosis in workplaces: how knowledgeable are the workers in Bangladesh? BMC Public Health 2015; 15(1): 1291.
[http://dx.doi.org/10.1186/s12889-015-2622-4] [PMID: 26703074]

[2]     Wong A, Marrie TJ, Garg S, Kellner JD, Tyrrell GJ. Welders are at increased risk for invasive pneumococcal disease. Int J Infect Dis 2010; 14(9): e796-9.
[http://dx.doi.org/10.1016/ j. ijid. 2010. 02.2268] [PMID: 20637673]

[3]     Molina-Gamboa JD, Poncr-de-Leon-Rosales S, Guerrero-Almeida ML, *et al.* Salmonella gastroenteritis outbreak among workers from a tertiary care hospital in Mexico City.ev. Invest Clin 199749(5): 349-53.

[4]     Ahmad A, Khan MU, Gogoi LJ, *et al.* Japanese Encephalitis in Assam, India: Need to increase healthcare workers' understanding to inprove health care. PLoS One 2015; 10(8): e0135767.
[http://dx.doi.org/10.1371/journal.pone.0135767] [PMID: 26296212]

[5]     Undeğer U, Başaran N, Kars A, Güç D. Assessment of DNA damage in nurses handling antineoplastic drugs by the alkaline COMET assay. Mutat Res 1999; 439(2): 277-85.
[http://dx.doi.org/10.1016/S1383-5718(99)00002-9] [PMID: 10023083]

[6]     Sari-Minodier I, Orsiere T, Auquier P, *et al.* Cytogenic monitoring by the use of micronucleus assay among hospital workers exposed to low doses of ionizing radiation. Mutant Res 2007; 629(2): 111-21.

[7]     Skov T, Maarup B, Olsen J, *et al.* Leukemia and reproductive outcome among nurses handling antineoplastic drugs. Br Ind Med 1992; 49(12): 855-61.

[8]     Shen CC, Hu YW, Hu LY, *et al.* The risk of cancer among Taiwansese female registered nurses: A nationwide retrospective study. PLoS One 2013; 8(7): e68420.
[http://dx.doi.org/10.1371/journal.pone.0068420] [PMID: 23874621]

[9]     Ribeiro T, Ribeiro T, Ribeiro T. Serranheiraf, Loureiro H. Work related musculoskeletal disorders in primary health care nurses. Appl Nurs Res 2017; 3372-7.

[10]    Chodick G, Bekiroglu N, Hauptmann M, *et al.* Risk of cataract after exposure to low doses of ionizing radiation: A 20-year prospective cohort study among US radiologic technologists. Am J Epidemiol 2008; 168(6): 620-31.
[http://dx.doi.org/10.1093/aje/kwn171] [PMID: 18664497]

[11]    Durán A, Hian SK, Miller DL, Le Heron J, Padovani R, Vano E. Recommendations for occupational radiation protection in interventional cardiology. Catheter Cardiovasc Interv 2013; 82(1): 29-42.
[http://dx.doi.org/10.1002/ccd.24694] [PMID: 23475846]

[12]    Shin JM, Lee TH, Park SH, *et al.* A survey of the radiation exposure protection of healthcare providers during endoscopic retrograde Cholangiopancreatography in Korea. Gut Liver 2013; 7(1): 100-5.
[http://dx.doi.org/10.5009/gnl.2013.7.1.100] [PMID: 23422932]

[13]    Churchyard GJ, Chaisson RE, Maartens S, *et al.* Tuberculosis preventive therapy to reduce individual risk of Tb and contribute to TB control. S Afr Med J 2014; 104(5): 339-43.
[http://dx.doi.org/10.7196/SAMJ.8290] [PMID: 25212199]

[14]    Edlich RF, Wind TC, Heather CL, *et al.* Recommendations for postexposure prophylaxis of operating room personnel and patients exposed to bloodborne diseases. J Long Term Eff Med Implants 2003; 12(2): 103-16.
[http://dx.doi.org/10.1615/JLongTermEffMedImplants.v13.i2.50] [PMID: 14510284]

CHAPTER 5

# Biosafety Issues for Scientists and Laboratory Workers

**Achla Gupta[1,*]** and **Farhana Zahir[2]**

[1] *Department of Pharmacological Sciences, Ichan School of Medicine at Mount Sinai, New York, NY10029, USA*

[2] *Prism Educational Society, Aligarh, U.P., India*

**Abstract:** A lab worker was severely burned working with a bottle of t-butyl-lithium. Tertiary butyl-lithium is a highly volatile chemical and spontaneously catches fire upon exposure to air. A scientist died working with bacteria; the infection that killed the scientist may be connected to a virus that causes small pox. Accidents in academic settings happen quite frequently every year in developed and developing countries. Most of the time, laboratories are fully stocked with hazardous chemicals such as strong acids, flammable items and neurotoxins. They also have natural gas-guzzling Bunsen burners and high-pressure cookers called autoclaves. Additionally, biology labs often have infectious organisms, chemistry labs have explosives, and physics labs often have lasers. Factually, everywhere you turn, there is something that could seriously injure you. But we cannot stop them from working on those things which improve the health of mankind. On the other hand, we have to take precautions in the laboratory for safe handling of biological materials and living organisms. The primary purpose of this chapter is to learn work safely with biological materials as well as to address other issues such as knowledge of specific biological agents and toxins, quality laboratory management practices and an overall safety culture.

**Keywords:** Biosafety Levels1 (BSL-1), Biosafety Level 2 (BSL-2), Biosafety Levels 3 (BSL-3), Biosafety Level 4 (BSL-4), Biosecurity, Bloodborne Pathogens, Bloodborne Diseases, Chemical Waste, Facility Construction, General Laboratory Safety, Genetically Modified Organisms (Gmos), Hepatitis B (HBV),Human Immunodeficiency Virus (HIV), Research Animal Waste, Radiation Waste, Safety Equipment, Transgenic Plants, Transgenic And "Knock-Out" Animals, Viral Vectors For Gene Transfer, Waste Disposal.

## What is Biosafety?

Recent years have seen quantum leap in medical biotechnology and biomedical

---

* **Corresponding author Achla Gupta:** Department of Pharmacological Sciences, Ichan School of Medicine at Mount Sinai, New York, NY 10029, USA.; Email: achla.gupta@mssm.edu

**Farhana Zahir (Ed.)**

engineering. Both the fields require handling of sensitive materials like pathogens (bacteria, virus, rickettsiae, fungi, prions), genetically modified plants/animals for the purpose of identification, improvement of trait or vaccine production, therapeutic intervention, *etc.* besides research, training and teaching. The increased interaction with the highly sensitive materials for any of the above-stated purposes may give rise to laboratory-acquired infections. The work of Edward Jenner (1749-1828), Loius Pasteur (1822-1895) and Robert Koch (1843-1910) contributed vastly towards understanding the principles of infectious diseases. Jenner discovered vaccination; Pasteur discovered the significance of sterilization in preventing the infection and germ theory of disease. Koch gave famous postulates of disease. The work of numerous scientists over subsequent years established progression of knowledge that confirmed connection between human pathogens, disease and preventive methods. Biosafety is a set of procedures laid down to safeguard not only scientists and laboratory workers but also the environment from potentially infectious microorganisms and other biological hazards.

There is no systematic survey to calculate the approximate number of laboratory acquired infections by scientists worldwide. According to a report published in 1995, an estimated 500,000 workers in the United States are at risk of laboratory-related infections ranging from severe to harmless [1]. The ever increasing workload on laboratories demand dedicated studies in order to safeguard the health of a laboratory worker. In any case, the risk of laboratory acquired infection is higher than that of the general public. According to a study published on laboratory acquired infections in Asia –Pacific region, only 27 reviews were found to be published between 1982-2016 [2], this report has no way to calculate the number of unpublished reports. The teaching laboratories, biological research laboratories, clinical and diagnostic laboratories, besides veterinary facilities, are places of human interface with potential human or animal tissue samples. It is a standard practice to have an ethical committee comprising of senior administrative members and senior scientists who supervise each and every aspect of the carefully designed experiment minimizing the associated risks to the laboratory worker or environment. It is the job of the committee to foresee if the laboratory meets standard prerequisites for the experiment while the laboratory in-charge ensures that his/her laboratory members follow every safety rule to the book.

**What are Biosafety Issues?**

Any issue associated with laboratory safety, whether it is **biological or chemical or radioactive** in **origin** that creates any health or environmental concern, **immediate or long-term**, is discussed under Biosafety issues. Issues of biological origin include blood-borne pathogens (BBP) including parasites, viruses and bacteria, recombinant DNA (rDNA), genetically modified organisms/crops, biological waste disposal, infectious substance and diagnostic specimen shipping (Fig. **1**). A lot of information is available over biosafety issues but third world countries like Pakistan show poor awareness levels on issues like vaccination, blood disposal, needle- handling, needle stick injury *etc.,* [3]. They also lack basic laboratory facilities.

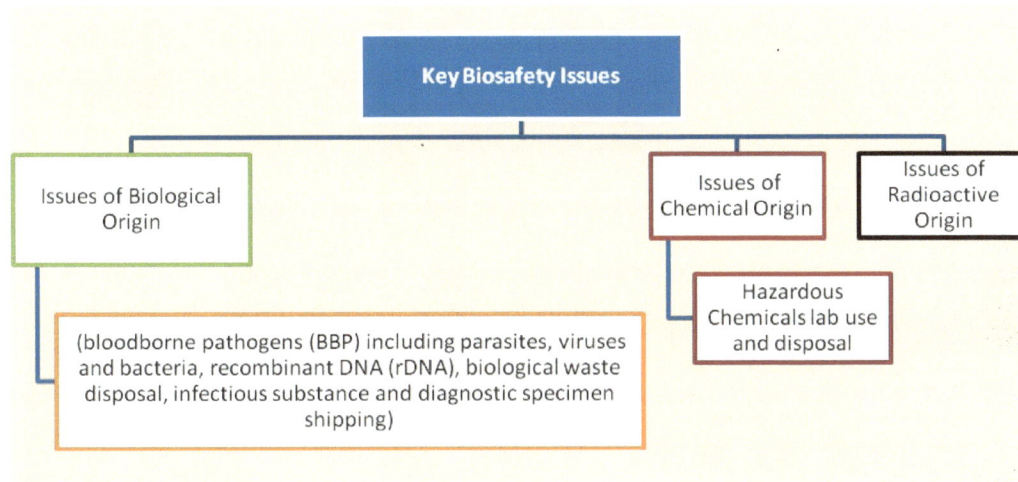

**Fig. (1).** Key Biosafety Issues.

## *Laboratory Safety*

All the safety issues, procedures, precautions and apprehensions related to the technical and non–technical staff working in the laboratory and institute are discussed under Laboratory Safety. Every head of the institute must respond to the anticipated laboratory safety issues which may arise during the experiment before allowing any new project and continuously review whether ongoing investigations are following safety procedures. Any lapse in the laboratory safety may turn out to be a biological hazard for the Institute personnel at micro level and the area in the vicinity of the institute at the macro level. The source of the risk could be biological (example: deadly virus/blood), chemical (example: DDT), radiological or laser *etc.,* or combination; depending on the nature of work conducted in the various laboratories of the same institute. Every laboratory has standard operating procedures besides, biological safety issues they include proper hazardous waste management disposal and drainage, emergency spill or accident response [4]. The commonly available laboratory tools like compressed gas cylinders, chemical fume hood/laminar flow, centrifuges as well as biological safety cabinets also need expert handling.

## Common Laboratory Care Practices (Fig. 2)

**1(a). Maintenance (Cleanliness):** The laboratory should be kept clean daily by ensuring proper disposal of waste, discarding used absorbent pads, pipette tips, needles, broken glassware, syringes *etc.* and wiping bench tops clean. Meticulous housekeeping requires detailed cleaning of the cabinets and refrigerators and deep freezers at least once a week; any damaged samples should be discarded. There should be a place for everything and everything in place to optimize the use of space and time in laboratory. All unnecessary glassware should be kept inside cabinets after thorough cleaning. The floors should be kept free of boxes, instruments and supplies by storing them properly. Keeping the laboratory clean goes a long way by avoiding accidents, spills, falls *etc.*

**(b) Maintenance (Electricity):** The electrical load of the laboratory should be calculated, and the use of electricity should not at any time exceed the allocated wattage. The facility should be provided with proper earthing (grounding) systems and fuses. Concealed electrical connections to sinks and water outlets are essential safety measures. Besides, the faulty wires, cables, thermostats, switch boards should

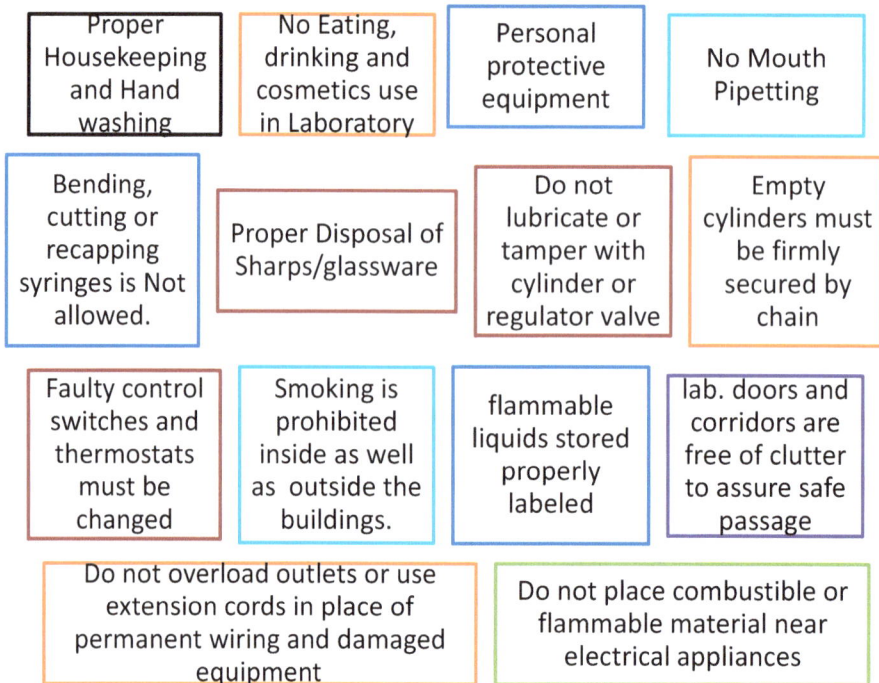

| | | | |
|---|---|---|---|
| Proper Housekeeping and Hand washing | No Eating, drinking and cosmetics use in Laboratory | Personal protective equipment | No Mouth Pipetting |
| Bending, cutting or recapping syringes is Not allowed. | Proper Disposal of Sharps/glassware | Do not lubricate or tamper with cylinder or regulator valve | Empty cylinders must be firmly secured by chain |
| Faulty control switches and thermostats must be changed | Smoking is prohibited inside as well as outside the buildings. | flammable liquids stored properly labeled | lab. doors and corridors are free of clutter to assure safe passage |
| Do not overload outlets or use extension cords in place of permanent wiring and damaged equipment | | Do not place combustible or flammable material near electrical appliances | |

**Fig. (2).** Rules for General Laboratory Safety.

be immediately replaced. It is not advisable to use extension cord in laboratory. **The ill-functioning equipment must never be used.**

**2. Personal protective kit**: A laboratory coat or smock and disposable gloves are essential for scientists or laboratory workers while at work in a laboratory. The other items of the protective kit might be chemical aprons, splash goggles, masks, face shields or respirators *etc.* according to the work carried out in the laboratory. The tools of the kit should be used appropriately.

**Gloves** (Fig. **3**) are worn while working with alkali, acid, blood, infectious or potentially hazardous/radioactive material. Gloves comprise the most widely used form of individual protective equipment as *they serve as a crucial barrier between the hands and unwanted materials.* Therefore, they should be chosen with great care depending on their thickness, concentration of solution (A strong acidic solution might need sturdy gloves), time duration of wearing, temperature at which work is going to be carried out, penetration capability of sharps and above all, reactivity with a particular chemical that is going to be used after wearing them. Simple **Latex gloves** were most common hand protection gears for a worker due to durability, low cost, touch sensitivity, fitness for most biological and aqueous radioactive work. However, these days, latex gloves come coated with disinfectant and recent decades have discovered that some people are allergic to latex. Latex sensitivity may range from mild itching to severe asthma or drop in blood pressure. Therefore, now-a-days, **Nitrile gloves** are used as an alternative to latex. Nitrile gloves are more expensive than Latex gloves. Generally, gloves go well with organic acids. Most inorganic acids get protection with Viton. Latex reacts very quickly with acids like Sulphuric acid and chromic acid and alkalis like ammonium hydroxide besides alcohols and amines, phenols, acrylamide, nitro benzene, acetic anhydride and Picric acid *etc.* Hence, latex gloves should not be used when these chemicals are worked with. Most glove materials like latex, neoprene, butyl, PVC are not suitable to work with aromatic hydrocarbons, aliphatic hydrocarbons, halogenated hydrocarbons, and esters. The exception to the list is butyl gloves; they are good to work with most esters, aldehydes and ketones. Neoprene is good to work while working with glycols. Viton gloves should be used while working with most halogens and mercury. Now- a-days, the glove suppliers give data on the glove safety depending on its stability, reactivity and permeability of its material; it should be consulted for specificity purposes. **Double gloving is recommended while doing surgery to prevent injury from sharps and handling extremely toxic substances like dimethyl mercury. According to the EN 374 European standard, gloves should have a 'microorganism' pictogram indicating that the gloves conform to at least performance level 2 for penetration test.**

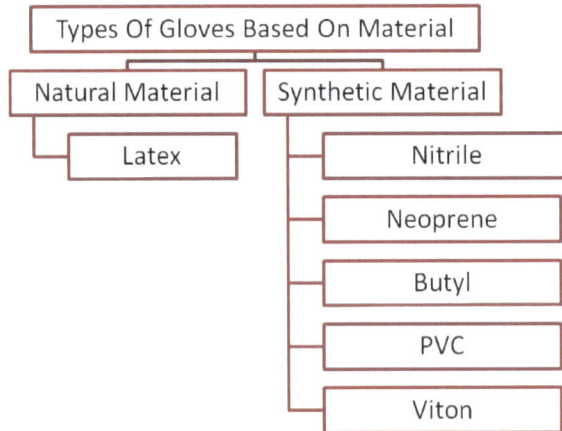

**Fig. (3).** Types of gloves based on synthesis material.

- The gloves should be used while transporting/cleaning radioactive or hazardous materials besides doing routine laboratory work
- Do not re-use disposable gloves; moreover, check for any holes or discoloration before wearing. Also check expiry date.
- Always use ungloved hand to help opening doors, pressing elevator buttons *etc.*
- Hands should be washed immediately after removal of gloves.
- Do not unintentionally touch the face or eyes while working with gloved hand, it might carry any potential toxic or infectious material. For similar reasons, do not touch mobile/cellphone, computer keyboard or any electric device or go out of laboratory area before removing contaminated gloves and washing hands.
- Disposable glove material is easily flammable. Ensure appropriate safety measures while going near high temperature sources.

**3. Pipetting:** Mechanical pipetting aids must be used when pipetting any material. Mouth pipetting is not allowed at any containment level.

**4. Syringes and Pasteur pipettes:** Exposed needles must be carefully disposed in the special sharps containers. Bending, cutting or recapping syringes is **not allowed**. Do not try to re-sheath needles or remove them from syringe as these manipulations can easily result in accidents.

**5. Broken Glassware:** All broken glassware must be placed in the sharps containers using tongs, dustpan, heavy gloves and broom. These sharps containers should be located within the lab.

**Waste and spills:** All infectious waste must be autoclaved or decontaminated before throwing in biological trash can. Care must be taken to generate minimum amount of aerosol. A general record of all major spills/accidents should be maintained.

**6. Gas cylinders:** Lab workers should be careful while working with compressed gas cylinders. Do not lubricate or tamper with cylinder or regulator valve. Proper regulators must be used. All compressed gas cylinders including empty cylinders must be firmly secured by chain to the wall or bench all the time.

**7. Electrical Equipment:** High voltage electrical equipment must be periodically checked by the Maintenance Department of the institution. These equipment should be labeled properly. Never ever try to by-pass the ground or safety devices on a piece of electrical equipment. Because it is too dangerous for the environment. Faulty control switches and thermostats must be changed immediately by the maintenance department.

**8. Fire Safety:** Fire safety is very essential element to any institution. All scientists or laboratory workers should know about these basic rules to prevent fire in working area.

- The foremost important rule: Smoking is **prohibited** inside as well as outside the buildings.
- Do not allow trash to accumulate in working area and always use the proper trash receptacles.
- Always remember to store flammable liquids properly in a cabinet labeled flammable items and keep combustible items to minimum in your work area.
- Make sure laboratory doors and corridors are free of clutter to assure safe passage in the event of an emergency.
- Electrical safety is very important to eliminate fire risks. For that, do not overload outlets, do not use extension cords in place of permanent wiring and damaged equipment. Always remember not to place combustible or flammable material near electrical appliances that produce heat.

However, even with a good program of prevention, fire occurring still exists. In that case, always remember **R.U.N** (Fig. **4**).

- **R-** Raise alarm, call emergency fire department.
- **U-**Unlock windows and doors and unplug working electronic equipment or any burner.
- **N-**Never forget to inform other laboratory personnel or support staff working in near you.
- All personnel, upon employment, should know where the nearest location of the fire alarm (usually located near fire exits) is and how to use it as well as where the extinguisher and how to use it, as well as the location of the extinguisher and

how to use it. **Class ABC extinguisher is best to prevent all types of fire**. You can use this extinguisher on combustibles (wood, paper), solvents, gasoline, oils and electrical. Always remember not to let the fire get between you and the exit (and alternative exit) and also know eye wash station, safety shower and how to use it.

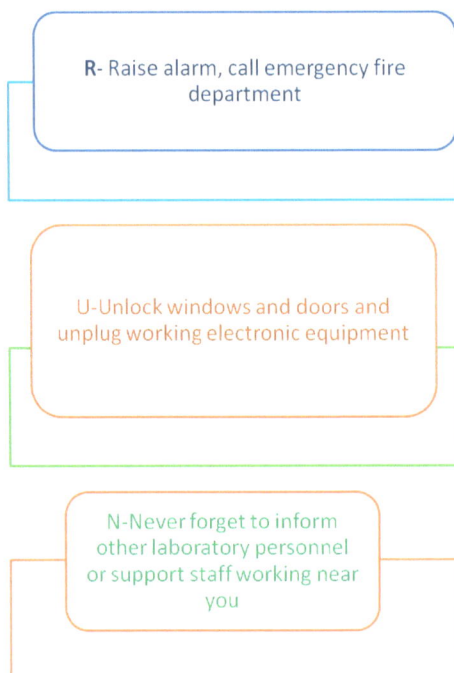

**R**- Raise alarm, call emergency fire department

U-Unlock windows and doors and unplug working electronic equipment

N-Never forget to inform other laboratory personnel or support staff working near you

**Fig. (4).** R.U.N.The three steps to remember during a fire outbreak.

9. **Eating, drinking, cosmetics and clothes:** The areas where bio-hazardous materials like infectious/radioactive/chemical carcinogens are used or stored should always prohibit eating or drinking. Smoking, chewing gum/tobacco, application of cosmetics, combing hair, shaving and brushing of teeth are other banned practices in lab. Storage of food/water/drink meant for human consumption is forbidden in laboratory refrigerators or freezers. **No Food or Drink** sign should be pasted on all refrigerators housing biological, chemical or radioactive substances. Always store laboratory coats, overalls separately to avoid contamination probably in cupboard outside the laboratory.

10. **Hazard Warnings:** All laboratory equipment, reagents and containers (*i.e.* flasks, beakers bottles and test tube) used for different purposes must be labeled appropriately. For example, if you are working with radioactive material that bench should be labeled with radioactive sign as well as the instruments also.

Storage cabinets, refrigerators, cold rooms, incubators, *etc.* all must be clearly identified with appropriate labels, signs, or other conspicuous identification. The exterior surface of laboratory doors should be reserved for hazard communication and appropriate purpose only. These are some general principles for laboratory safety. However, there is more to know about the biological agents. Biological agents, plants or animals are classified according to biosafety level risk groups (Table **1**). These classifications presume ordinary circumstances in the research laboratory, or growth of agents in small volumes for diagnostic and experimental purposes. These biological agents are potentially infectious microbes and limit contamination of the work environment and the community. Bio-containment can be classified by the relative danger to the surrounding environment as biological safety levels (BSL).

## What are Biosafety Levels (BSLs)

Biosafety is the use of security measures that reduces the risk of exposure of any pathogen to a scientist from potential biological toxins carrying tissues like blood or transgenic therapy products/genetic material or infective organisms like bacteria, fungi, viruses, parasites in order to save the researcher, laboratory worker, staff, patient, community and the ecosystem from the unwanted consequences of the biological leakage.

There are four biosafety levels depending on the level of biological risk assessment (Table **1**).

Risk group 1: Very low or negligible individual and community risk

Risk group 2: Moderate individual and community risk

Risk group 3: High individual and community risk

Risk group 4: Extremely high individual and community risk.

Each level has specific controls for containment of microbes and biological agents. The primary risks that determine levels of containment are infectivity, severity of disease, transmissibility, and the nature of the work conducted. Origin of the microbe and the route of exposure are also important while deciding the category of laboratory. The requirement of laboratory Isolation (ease of public access), ventilation (HEPA/directional), double door entry, anteroom (with/without shower), air lock (with/without shower), autoclave (single/double), biosafety cabinet (I, II, III) and effluents treatment are certain parameters which are taken under consideration depending on the desirable biosafety level (Fig. **5**). The risk group 1 requires a biosafety level 1 laboratory or BSL-1 laboratory.

Similarly, risk group 2 requires a biosafety level 2 laboratory or BSL-2, risk group 3 requires a biosafety level 3 laboratory or BSL-3, risk group 4 requires a biosafety level 4 laboratory or BSL-4. Each biosafety level builds on the controls of the level before it [5, 6] in terms of facility construction, safety equipment and laboratory practices (Fig. **6**). Every biology laboratory, regardless of biosafety level, follows standard microbiological practices. Standard microbiological practices are those practices that are common to all laboratories. These practices have been briefly discussed in section 1.1.

Biological safety cabinets are an important laboratory safety device. They are crucially used in detection and identification of pathogens in laboratories worldwide. The purchase, use and maintenance of Biological safety cabinets is compromised in low and middle income countries. Hands on training on repair, maintenance and proper use of biological safety cabinets is available [7].

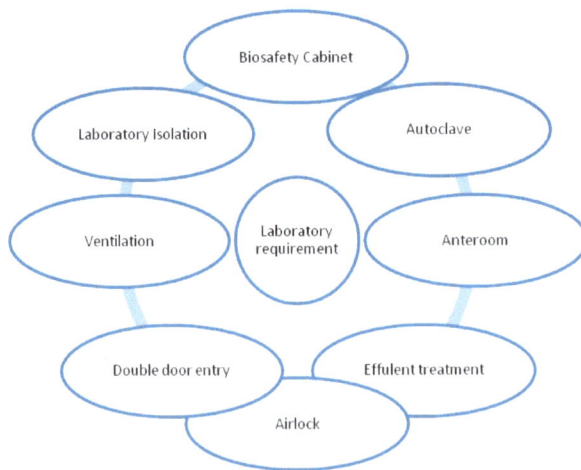

Fig. (5). Parameter checklist for a functional laboratory depending on biosafety level.

## Biosafety Level 1 (BSL-1)

BSL-1 (Table **1**) is suitable for work concerning well-characterized agents or microbes not known to consistently cause disease in healthy adult humans. They present minimal potential hazard to laboratory workers and the environment and hence, are usually located in colleges for the purpose of basic teaching. It includes several kinds of bacteria and viruses including nonpathogenic *Escherichia coli*, as well as some cell cultures and non-infectious bacteria. BSL-1 laboratories are not necessarily segregated (Fig. **5**) from the general public in the building. Laboratory personnel must have specialized training in the procedures conducted in the

laboratory. Specific considerations for a BSL-1 laboratory include the following:

## Laboratory Practices

- Standard microbiological practices are followed.
- Work can be performed on an open bench.
- Personal protective equipment (PPE) like gloves worn to minimize exposure.

## Facility Construction

- A sink must be available for hand washing.
- The laboratories should have separate and easily cleanable working space.
- Bench tops must be resistant to water, heat, organic solvents, acids, alkalis and other chemicals.
- *Furniture should be selected for ease of cleaning and decontamination.

**Table 1. Risk Group Classification.**

| Risk Group 1 | Risk Group 2 | Risk Group 3 | Risk Group 4 |
|---|---|---|---|
| Agents are not associated with disease in healthy adult humans (Low risk). | Agents are associated with human disease which is rarely serious. There are often preventive or therapeutic interventions available. (Moderate risk) | Agents are associated with serious or lethal human or animal disease but does not ordinarily spread from one infected individual to another. Effective treatment and preventive measures are available. | Agents are likely to cause serious or lethal human disease and that can be readily transmitted from one individual to another, directly or indirectly. Effective treatment and preventive measures are not usually available (Extreme risk) |
| Examples: Escherichia coli; K12 derivatives (DH5a, JH109, pBluescript, psi2) | Examples: Adenovirus all types, All human blood contaminated specimens; HIV/SIV infected animals. Human cell lines eg. HEK 293, HeLa , Herpes Simplex Virus, Rabies Virus. | Risk Group 3 has high individual risk and low community risk | Risk Group 4 has high individual and community risk |
| | | Example: chickungunya, rickettsia, SARS Corona Virus | Example: Nipah virus, Marburg virus, variolla (small pox) |

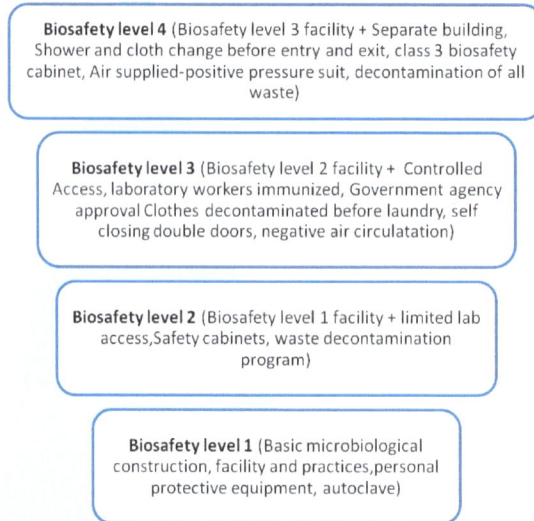

**Fig. (6).** Safety measures increase as the biosafety level increases; highest for Biosafety level 4 and lowest for Biosafety level 1.

**Fig. (7).** Comparison of biosafety level 1 and 2.

## Biosafety Level 2 (BSL-2)

This level can be built by upgrading a BSL-1 facility. The typical BSL-2 microbes are spread through ingestion, inhalation or percutaneous injury causing ailments of varying severity; posing moderate hazards to laboratory workers and the environment. These microbes are common for the geographic region. This level includes bacteria and viruses that cause only mild diseases to humans, or are difficult to acquire through aerosol in a lab. setting, such as *Staphylococcus aureus*, *C. difficile*, most *Chlamydiae*, *hepatitis A, B,* and *C*, orthopoxviruses (other than smallpox), influenza A, lyme disease, Salmonella, mumps, measles *etc.* The BSL-2 laboratories have the following containment requirements (Fig. **7**).

## Laboratory Practices

- Restricted access to the laboratory during working hours.
- Suitable personal protective equipment (PPE) is worn, including laboratory coats and gloves. Appropriate respirators, eye protection and face shields can also be worn, as needed.
- All procedures are performed within a biological safety cabinet (BSC). Biosafety cabinets are specially designed to protect the worker from infectious aerosols.
- An autoclave or an alternative method of decontamination like chemical disinfection or incineration must be used.

## Facility Construction

- The laboratory has self-closing doors.
- A sink and eye wash are readily available to physically wash the eyes in case of contamination.

## Biosafety Level 3 (BSL-3)

BSL-3 (Fig. **8**) can be built by upgrading BSL-2 laboratory. This level includes all clinical and diagnostic research laboratories as the investigations with indigenous or exotic agents may lead to deadly diseases like tuberculosis through respiratory transmission. It also contains various bacteria, parasites and viruses such as *Mycobacterium tuberculosis, Chlamydia psittaci, Coxiella burnetii, Eastern equine encephalitis virus, Rickettsia rickettsii*, several species of *Brucella*, rabies virus, yellow fever virus, and West Nile virus that can cause severe to fatal disease in humans but for these diseases, treatment is available. In addition to BSL-2 facility, BSL-3 laboratories have the following compulsory requirements.

## Laboratory Practices

- The people working in these laboratories are under medical surveillance and might receive immunizations for microbes they work with. It is a pre-requisite that the laboratory workforce has specialized guidance in handling pathogenic and potentially lethal agents, and the laboratory operations are under the aegis of competent scientists with prior experience [8]. Moreover, the workers particularly women of childbearing age should be informed of dangers of working in such an environment.

- Due to biosecurity reasons no person is ever allowed to work alone in this laboratory.
- Hand washing procedures must be implanted strictly.
- Any accidents must be immediately reported to responsible staff.
- Extra care should be taken during collection/handling of infectious material. It must be stored in leak/spill proof packing.
- Decontamination of waste should be performed before transport in accordance with the legal framework of the country. **A detailed safety manual must be developed according to the work conducted in the laboratory and strictly implemented.**
- All time restricted admission to the laboratory.

## Safety Equipment

- All procedures are conducted within appropriate biological safety cabinets (Class II) or specially designed hoods.
- Specialized PPE for BSL-3 laboratory includes laboratory coats and gowns which open at the back and separate laboratory shoes with covers. **Laboratory clothing must be decontaminated before disposal or laundry**; whichever is applicable.
- Respirators must be worn all the time when you are working in BSL-3 laboratories including animal house. Respirator is a kind of equipment which covers the nose and mouth or the entire face or head. Lab. respirators filter out infectious or harmful particles; some supply the wearer with HEPA-filtered air. Appropriate respirators are chosen based on the type of work being performed.

## Facility Construction

- The laboratory space is separate from the entire building with sealed windows and two sets of self-closing and locking doors.
- Sealed openings are provided to facilitate decontamination.
- A hands-free sink and eyewash are available near the exit.
- Exhaust air cannot be re-circulated, and the laboratory must have sustained directional airflow by drawing air into the laboratory from clean areas towards potentially contaminated areas. The exhaust air must be discharged outside the building. HEPA filters are installed in a manner to ease gaseous decontamination of air.

| Biosafety Level 3 (BSL-3) | Biosafety Level 4 (BSL-4) |
|---|---|
| • Works on serious or potentially lethal diseases for which treatment is available.<br>• Laboratory practices: BSL-2 + practices, PPE and respirators are MUST, HEPA-filtered air. workers under medical surveillance, immunizations and Entry is restricted.<br>• Facility construction: : BSL-2 + construction ,Exhaust air cannot be re-circulated, two sets of self-closing and locking doors.<br>• Example: Mycobacterium tuberculosis, all Clinical and diagnostic research laboratories. | • Works on dangerous diseases for which NO treatment is available.<br>• Laboratory practices: BSL-3 + practices, Class III biological safety cabinets, Highly specialized garments  worn before entering, Shower upon exiting, decontamination of all materials before exiting, Trained scientists Enter inside only by permission.<br>• Facility construction: restricted zone of the building, use negatively pressurized facilities, dedicated supply and exhaust air,  vacuum lines and decontamination systems, Multiple airlocks prevent opening of both doors at  same time.<br>• Example: Marburg Virus . |

**Fig. (8).** Comparison of biosafety level 3 and 4.

## Biosafety Level 4 (BSL-4)

BSL-4 (Fig. **8**) is the top most level of biological safety; hence the laboratory is delineated from the main building. These laboratories come directly under state control due to nature of high risk work conducted here. The microbes in a BSL-4 lab are dangerous and exotic, posing highest risk of aerosol-transmitted infections. Infections caused by these microbes are frequently fatal and without known treatment or vaccines.

There are only a few BSL-4 labs around the world. **Centers for Disease Control and Prevention** (United States), **Atlanta Swedish Institute for Communicable Disease Control** (Sweden),**Centre for Cellular and Molecular Biology** (India), **Bernhard Nocht Institute for Tropical Medicine** (Germany), **National Institute for Communicable Diseases** (Africa), **Virology Laboratory of the Queensland Department of Health** (Australia) are a few famous BSL-4 laboratories currently operating in the world. The examples of microbes worked within a BSL-4 laboratory include Nipah and Marburg viruses. They are considered dangerous enough to require the additional safety measures, regardless of vaccination availability. The BSL-4 laboratory is built upon the containment requirements of BSL-3 laboratory after much deliberation with experienced scientists.

**Safety Equipment**: There can be two types of BSL-4 labs or a combined laboratory.

a. **Class III cabinet laboratory:** The Class III biological cabinet laboratories have a dedicated shower with changing rooms for workers. Any material/supply entering/exiting the cabinet is either autoclaved or fumigated.

b. **Suit laboratory:** One-piece suits have positive pressure with HEPA filters and independent emergency air supply. The suits have all facilities of a Class III biological cabinet.

## Laboratory Practices

- Change of clothing is mandatory before entry and exit.
- Entry and exit is through air lock system.
- All the waste and effluents should be decontaminated and the pH of the effluent must be neutralized.
- The air is also decontaminated before leaving in order to prevent any accidental release of pathogens.
- These laboratories have policies for avoiding use of sharps like syringes and needles except in cases with no alternative. In case of broken glassware, extreme precautions are taken; they are never touched by hand.
- All laboratory workers should have specific and thorough training in handling extremely hazardous infectious agents. They should have the knowledge of the primary and secondary containment functions of the standard and special practices, the containment equipment, and the laboratory design characteristics. Only qualified scientists who are trained and experienced in working with these agents should work in BSL-4 laboratories.
- Access to the laboratory is strictly controlled by the laboratory director. All time restricted admission to the laboratory is to be maintained.
- A specific facility operations manual is prepared or adopted. Building protocols for preventing contamination often use negatively pressurized facilities, which, even if compromised, would severely inhibit an outbreak of aerosol pathogens.
- All operations are conducted in conformation with the laws of the country. In case of accidental fire, police and medical emergency numbers should be immediately called.

## Facility Construction

- The laboratory is in a separate building or in an isolated and restricted zone of the building.
- The construction design ensures dedicated supply of air and the whole laboratory has well maintained negative air pressure.

- Multiple airlocks with electronic security are engaged to prevent both doors from opening at the same time. Besides showers, a vacuum room, an ultraviolet light room, and other safety measures are installed to wipe out all the traces of biohazard.
- Exhaust air lines, vacuum lines and decontamination systems are also installed to prevent infection.

## Biosafety from Pathogens

Scientists and laboratory workers are under constant threat due to their high risk occupation. Besides chemical and radiation hazards, working in a biomedical laboratory exposes the worker to various pathogens. The pathogen may be partially known or fully known or completely unknown. Laboratory personnel work on all aspects from identification of the pathogen to making kits for easy identification besides searching for therapeutic interventions for treatment/prevention like vaccines. Different pathogens have varying virulence, incubation period and mode of transmission. Ingestion (through mouth pipetting or putting contaminated articles like pencil in mouth or consumption of eatables in laboratory), inoculation (through cuts, sharps and insect bite), inhalation (through aerosols), are key modes of infection besides spills, splashes and contaminated surfaces which come in contact with skin and membranes of organs like eyes. However, several unknown causes of infection in some cases are also expected [2].

**The causative agents of some infections overlap in symptoms and mimic identification tests. Therefore, at times, it becomes very difficult to identify the microbe to initiate treatment.** It is worth mentioning that high risk infections like anthrax and plague requiring high dose per infection are contained within laboratories with personal protective measures and availability of biosafety cabinets while infections requiring low dose like Q fever, tularemia, venezuelan equine encephalitis are contained only after the laboratory workers receive vaccination [9]. Additional challenges, besides the safety of the laboratory worker particularly in BSL 3 and 4 laboratories, are listed below:

1. Re-emerging infections like tuberculosis with resistant strains.
2. Infectious pathogens if accidently escape from workplace (laboratory) can threaten community health.
3. Laboratories working on pathogens of low dose high risk infectious agents require proper surveillance and need to maintain secrecy as they can be used as biological threat weapons.

## Biosafety from Bloodborne Pathogens

The Bloodborne Pathogen program was designed to lay foundation for organizations/institutions to build a strategy to provide data and awareness for basic learning of bloodborne pathogens and their common modes of transmission. Besides promoting deeper understanding of the implications of biosafety, the program has agenda to impart knowledge, training and technology to shield individuals from occupational exposures to blood or other potentially infectious materials.

## What are Bloodborne Pathogens?

**Bloodborne pathogens (BBP)** are viruses or bacteria or parasites; these microorganisms are carried in blood and can cause disease when transferred from an infected person to a healthy person through blood or other potentially infected body fluids. Infectious body fluids include amniotic fluid, cerebrospinal fluid, semen, vaginal secretions, synovial fluid, pleural fluid, peritoneal fluid, saliva in dental procedure, any fluid visibly contaminated with blood. It also includes any unfixed tissues or organ other than intact skin from a human (living or dead). Cell or tissue or organ cultures from experimental animals containing human immunodeficiency virus (HIV), Syphilis and Hepatitis B (HBV) are also considered as bloodborne pathogens. These microorganisms are capable of causing serious illness and death. Bloodborne diseases include malaria, Hepatitis C and Brucellosis *etc.* but **HBV** and **HIV** are the two diseases specifically addressed by **Occupational Safety and Health Administration (OSHA)**. In 1991, the OSHA established a Bloodborne Pathogens Program. The purpose of this program is to protect workers from the health hazards associated with bloodborne pathogens and to provide appropriate treatment and counseling should an employee be exposed to bloodborne pathogens. The OSHA standard applies only to human-human exposures unless the animal blood is used for research and is known to be infected with HIV or HBV {the Occupational Safety and Health Administration's (OSHA's) Bloodborne Pathogen Standard, 29 CFR 1910.1030}.

## How do Bloodborne Pathogens Spread in the Work Place?

Pathogens maybe introduced to laboratory personnel in multiple ways from clinical specimens, animals or vectors used in experiments, agents or aerosol generation.

a. Intact skin forms the foremost impervious barrier against bloodborne pathogens. Any sort of aperture or crack like open sores, cuts, abrasions, acne, any sort of damaged or broken skin such as sunburn or blisters *in the skin create a place for infected blood or fluids to enter the body of uninfected laboratory worker.* Needle stick injuries are the most common method of exposure for health care workers [10].

b. Bloodborne pathogens may also be transmitted through the mucous membranes of the eyes, nose and mouth. For example, a splash of contaminated blood to one's eyes, nose, or mouth could result in transmission. Non-laboratory workers may become exposed at work while providing help to an injured co-worker and coming in contact with the injured person's blood or body fluids. For example, if someone infected with HIV cut his/her finger on a piece of glass or puncture by needle and then you cut yourself on the now infected piece of glass or needle it is possible that you could contract the disease. Whenever there is blood-to-blood contact with infected blood or body fluid, it carries the risk of potential infection.

c. Aerosol generation is the most common procedure that often goes undetected. **Aerosols** are produced during laboratory procedures through routine activities like pipetting, blending, centrifugation, vortex mixing and sonicating *etc.* All these techniques lead to formation of air particles which remain suspended in air.

d. Other most common ways bloodborne pathogens spread are through sexual transmission or IV drug use.

However, if you have been involved in an exposure incident, stay calm, wash yourself thoroughly, and report to your supervisor right away. Inform your supervisor of how, when, where and whose blood you came in contact with and immediately seek medical attention. A medical professional will provide you with appropriate testing, treatment and education.

Some of the common laboratory acquired infections are listed below.

## Laboratory Acquired Bacterial Infections

**Brucella:** It is a very high risk infection reported to be transmitted through aerosol generation. Any minor lapse in safety measures results in disease in laboratory technicians. A laboratory worker acquired infection while harvesting live cells from a dog for antigen production [11]. Similarly, a report shows infection of a worker while taking aspirate from a patient in hospital outside laboratory [12]. Accidental breaking of a centrifuge tube resulted in illness of twelve laboratory workers in a lab in 1990, they were constantly monitored for symptoms and antibody titers for a period of year [13].

*N. meningitidis*: The first case of laboratory acquired meningococcal infection was reported from a field mobile laboratory world during world war I [14]. Meningitis, an infection of brain and spinal cord spreads easily if safety instructions are breached. A fatal meningitis case was reported from a California laboratory worker in 2012 due to violation of recommended safety regulations [15]. Regular use of personal protective equipment and vaccination has been reported to prevent the infection amongst laboratory workers as can be seen in European countries [16].

***Mycobacterium tuberculosis:*** It was in year 1993 that tuberculosis was declared a global emergency by world health organization. According to Center for Disease Control and prevention low infective dose of ≤10 bacilli is a cause of high rate of tuberculosis infection (2009); therefore, it is suggested that the laboratory procedures must be performed in class II biosafety cabinets. The laboratory workers have their own share of exposure due to human errors like accidental injection of Freund's complete adjuvant with mycobacterium tuberculosis [17] or exposure to pathogen during aerosol generation procedures like autopsy, culture, frozen sections *etc.* Unintentional exposure to the pathogen in high burden laboratories is a matter of concern [18]. All the preventive measures should be taken at the level of laboratory administration including proper training of workers, vaccination if required and constant availability of adequately functioning apparatus besides proper disposal of infective tissue, sputum, urine, stool, body fluids. The laboratory worker with suppressed immune system should be given preventive therapy regardless of tuberculin skin test result [19].

***Francisella tularensis:*** It is **class A** bioterrorism agent developed by USA and Soviet Union. Its ease of dispersal and high mortality rate triggers major public health concern making it a candidate bioterrorism agent. The laboratories should take special care as *Francisella tularensis* is often confused with *Hemophilus* species. Sometimes, it might also be mistaken for *Actinobacillus actinomycetemcomitans* or *Neisseria meningitides or Legionella pneumophila* due to overlapping reactions or symptoms. The aerosol generation procedures in laboratories or during autopsy often result in exposure to the organism due to delay in identification. An instance of fatal pulmonary tularemia of a 43-year-old man resulted in ***Francisella tularensis*** exposure despite presence of bioterrorism procedure [20]. The laboratory personnel were given doxycycline as a prophylactic measure.

***Bacillus anthracis:*** Bacillius was used as a bioterrorism agent against US in 2002 as envelopes containing spores were sent to the government officials threatening the most lethal disease form, pulmonary anthrax. There are three kinds of disease *viz*, cutaneous, gastrointestinal and pulmonary forms. It is difficult to identify pathogen in both vegetative and spore forms due to similarity in various bacillus species, although recently bioluminescent reporter phages have been used for rapid identification. *Cutaneous bacillus* was reported from a laboratory worker who had a cut and supported his colleague in carrying sample vials [21]. Therefore, laboratory workers should take all recommended precautions when dealing with suspected samples.

***Salmonella enterica:*** As it is a typical infection acquired from laboratory work, all routine precautions are undertaken to prevent it. Despite all biosafety measures, laboratory acquired infections do occur. Whole genome sequencing confirmed that a microbiologist from Saskatchewan Disease Control Laboratory (SDCL), Canada caught enterocolitis while working in a laboratory on *Salmonella enterica* [22]. This is noteworthy as a recent report concludes that severe salmonella infection manipulates signal transduction pathways and increases colon cancer risk [23].

***Salmonella typhi:*** There have been reports of laboratory acquired typhoid infections dating as far as 1961.It becomes difficult to identify the laboratory acquired typhoid, a class 3 infection caused by *Salmonella typhi* due to lack of characteristic symptoms [24]. Moreover, emerging strains require more than standard microbiological techniques. Advanced techniques like phage typing, antibiograms, pulse field gel electrophoresis, multilocus sequence typing and whole-genome sequencing (WGS) [25, 26].

**Shigella:** Infection has a high chance of becoming a laboratory epidemic if stringent safety precautions are ignored [27].

***Coxiella burnetii* induced Q fever:** Frequent records of laboratory infections from bacterium called *Coxiella burnetii* dating as far as 1935 are available. Low dose of infection required for Q fever makes it a subject of high risk research because it can be used as a biological weapon.

**Scrub Typhus:** It accounted for 32% laboratory acquired infections related deaths during 1931-2000 [28]. Any animal work or large scale culture work should be performed in high containment BSL 3 laboratory [28].

## Laboratory Acquired Viral Infections

**Dengue:** Dengue virus infection causing dengue fever has been reported from laboratory workers in Korea [10] and Japan [29] due to accidental needle stick injury. Out of 33% of occupational dengue infection, 24% was reported due to needle stick injury in Al-Madinah city [30]. **The high rate of infection in Asian continent suggests lack of biosafety training among workers and calls for stringent control measures on part of management to avert an avoidable infection.**

***Vaccinia virus* (VACV):** *Vaccinia virus* (VACV) is a potent pathogen causing ocular infections. It is a popular model organism used to study virus biology, host interaction, vaccine development *etc.* using non- highly attenuated viruses. A significant 28% vaccinia virus (VACV) infection causing conjunctivitis in laboratory workers was confirmed by DNA sequencing in Iran [31]. However, a case of infection in recently immunized laboratory worker makes it required to critically review the biosafety policy on *Vaccinia virus* [32].

**Small Pox:** It is a viral infection caused by *Variola virus.* It has been eradicated from the world. Today, small pox virus is present in laboratories for research purposes. OSHA (Occupational Safety and Health Administration) lists that small pox virus can be used as a bioweapon in the form of aerosol. It advises laboratory workers to follow standard precautions regarding contact and airborne diseases in suspected cases. **Advisory Committee on Immunization Practices(ACIP),** US recommends small pox vaccination for laboratory personnel who directly handles VACV (wild type Vaccinia virus). It recommends revaccination every 10 years for people working on non-highly attenuated VACV (*e.g.,* western reserve) or non-variola orthopox viruses, while people working on non-variola orthopoxviruses such as monkeypox are advised to be revaccinated every 3 years [32].

Other viral infections acquired during routine laboratory work include west Nile Virus [33], Hanta virus infection [34].

**Hepatitis:** Members of the families Picornaviridae, Hepadnaviridae, Flaviviridae and genus Delta, family **orthohepevirus B** are causative agents of **Hepatitis A (HAV), Hepatitis B (HBV), Hepatitis C (HCV), Hepatitis D (HDV) and Hepatitis E (HEV) viral** infections respectively. Laboratory infections of **Hepatitis A** (HAV) are reported among scientists working with induced or natural Hepatitis in chimpanzees while **Hepatitis B (HBV)** infection is reported from laboratory workers handling samples of human origin (National Academies Press – US, 1989). **Hepatitis B (HBV), Hepatitis C (HCV)** and **Hepatitis D (HDV)** viruses are other class 3 infections which may put the laboratory worker at risk to infection owing to needle stick injury or exposure to mucous membranes. Rhesus monkey, swine, chicken, rabbits, rats, ferrets and gerbils are used as experimental animal models for development of vaccine against **Hepatitis E (HEV).** The scientists need to take all precautions to prevent any accidental zoonotic infection. Although a vaccine against hepatitis A and B has been available since 1982, there are no human vaccines available for Hepatitis C, D and E. The currently available HBV vaccine is safe and effective in preventing 95% infection. The vaccine can be given as either three or four separate doses, as part of existing routine immunization schedules. Especially pregnant female scientists and laboratory workers should be given these vaccines if they are working with bloodborne pathogens where the hepatitis B virus is common to spread from mother-to-infant. *As HEV is a subviral satellite it can survive only in the presence of HBV, a vaccine for HBV works for HEV too.*

**Human Immunodeficiency Virus (HIV):** Acquired immune deficiency syndrome (AIDS) is caused by a virus called the Human Immunodeficiency Virus (HIV). This is a slowly-replicating lentivirus. Currently, there is no treatment for HIV/AIDS, other than a combination of drugs that are used to control the virus. Strict biosafety measures are required to be taken for this BSL-3 disease which primarily spreads through percutaneous and permucosal inoculation.

**Avian H5N1 Influenza:** It is a biosafety level 3 infection and hence, any work related to H5N1 should be conducted in biosafety cabinets. It generates aerosols very easily, thus high chance of infecting laboratory individuals. Therefore, they are advised to be proactive and prevent any aerosol generation [35].

**Laboratory Acquired Parasitic Infections**

Malaria, leishmaniasis, trypanosomiasis (African and American), and toxoplasmosis are some prominent laboratory acquired protozoal infections while there are only a few reports on laboratory acquired helminth infections barring a few schistosome cases. There have been numerous reports of parasitic infections from laboratory personnel primarily due to poor laboratory practices like sharp/needle stick injury, broken capillary, insect/animal bite, assuming that the organism was unviable or the strain does not affect humans [36].

**Biosafety for Recombinant-DNA (R-DNA)** Any modern biologist could not visualize to work without **Recombinant-DNA (R-DNA)** technology which includes combining genetic information from various sources consequently creating genetically modified organisms (GMOs) that may have never resided in natural world before. **Recombinant-DNA or** R-DNA technology has already had an enormous impact on fields like biology, medicine & pharmacy, agriculture and industrial biotechnology *etc.* Although it is a very functional technology giving us novel insights, tremendous applications, medical breakthroughs which are termed as **gain- of- function** (GOF) research, it involves potential pandemic pathogens (PPP) and genes of virulence which might be deliberately manipulated for misuse like enhanced virulence or disease resistance or transmission. WHO terms such research as **dual use research of concern (DURC).** Techniques like **CRISPR** have revolutionized health science as we witness first genetically edited human babies for flu resistance by Chinese scientists of the southern university of science and technology in the year 2018. But the same has become a subject of intense debate on moral and ethical grounds, amidst apprehensions about the misuse of technology. These developments have generated a sense of concern among molecular biologists that such organisms might have unpredictable and undesirable properties and would represent a biohazard if they escape from the laboratory. The visionaries of the scientific world could foresee these concerns and deliberated on the topic in the famous **Asilomar conference** held back more than four decades ago in 1975. At that meeting, safety issues were discussed and the first guidelines for R-DNA technology were proposed. In May 1976, **National Institutes of Health (NIH)** developed certain guidelines on R-DNA research. R-DNA advisory committee (RAC) was instituted in the same year to advise the director of NIH on issues of clinical trials involving recombinant DNA. Later, they added synthetic nucleic acid research to it. In 1980, clinical gene transfer studies also came under domain of RAC.NIH Guidelines for research involving Recombinant or Synthetic Nucleic Acid Molecules were implemented **through RAC** along with **Institutional Biosafety Committee (IBC) as the nodal agency for any recombinant DNA study based clinical trial or preclinical research**. The guidelines set down specific actions that include establishing safety procedures for R-DNA research, production and release to the environment and setting up containment conditions for certain experiments. In view of the research getting more advanced Institute of Medicine (IOM) has suggested that IBC should serve as the primary body to check compliance of the proposed experiments with NIH guidelines [37].

It was in '70s that the first time genetic engineering technology was used to clone human DNA segments of interest in bacterial hosts to produce insulin. The pharmaceutical production house, **Gentech** immediately saw merit in mass production of the insulin hormone. Gentech subsequently became the first molecular millionaire. The enthusiastic welcome by industry and scientists alike of the new technique opened unforeseen avenues for research and industry; the biotechnology or genetic engineering blossomed. Genetically modified higher organisms (GMO) such as transgenic and "knock-out" animals and transgenic plants have been created using R-DNA molecules. **All these developments have created renaissance in human and veterinary health, agriculture and environment science.** The general risks associated with recombinant DNA technology is possibility of undesirable display of genetic characteristics of donor and recipient organisms after fusion of DNA with hybrid vigour, taxonomy, identification, source and culture, pathogenic and physiological traits of donor and recipient organisms, and properties of the modified/engineered organism. Biosecurity issues are preventive measures according to the organism and techniques involved in the study. **Biosafety and biosecurity measures often overlap.** Biosafety issues for GMOs include handling, production, storing and transportation. Thus, **Cartagena protocol on biosafety** to the convention of biodiversity owes to protect biodiversity and human health from any risk emerging from GMO.

## Biological Expression Systems

Biological expression systems are vectors and host cells that fulfill a number of criteria that make them safe to use. All the facilities handling microorganisms and materials containing recombinant DNA molecules have risk assessment program. The risk assessment must consider not only the vector/host system used but also the properties of the DNA to be cloned. It includes nature, modification, function and source of the insert, stability of insert, vector construction, and transfer into host, frequency of mobilization, rate and level of expression, and influence of the recipient organism on the activity of the foreign protein. For example, biological agents such as *E. coli, S. cerevesiae, B. subtilis, etc.* are well characterized strains of microorganisms known to cause no disease in healthy adults. Thus, most routine genetic engineering experiments can be performed safely on *E. coli* K12/pUC18 at BSL-1. Mostly, the risk assessment will show that the inserted DNA sequences are unlikely to alter the biological properties of the host organism. However, if they are derived from a pathogenic organism they may alter the biological properties of the host organism. Obviously, not all genes of a pathogenic organism contribute to the virulence of the agent. Therefore, insertion of well-characterized DNA sequences that are unlikely to be involved in pathogenicity may not require additional safety measures. However, in cases where these sequences are not characterized, a higher BSL will be required. Though, cloning of genes coding for proteins such as toxins may thus require higher BSLs. When the gene product has potential pharmacological activity, then a higher BSL will be required. For example, overexpression of gene products from eukaryotic viral vectors can have unexpected consequences because these proteins have pharmacological activity. **However, scientists are working on microbial switches and biofirewalls based on molecular circuit based control of cell viability [38, 39]; they are designed to kill the bacteria if it accidently escapes controlled environment of a bacterial containment.**

## Vectors for Gene Transfer

Gene therapy has become a possible and efficient strategy for the treatment of both monogenetic and acquired diseases. Vectors, *in vivo* or *ex vivo* are used not only for gene therapy but also for efficient transfer of genes to other cells besides **immunomodulation**. The vectors may be viral or non-viral like DNA or DNA-protein complexes or liposomes. Non-viral vectors are preferred over viral vectors due to concerns over biosafety [40]. Any gene delivery method will have to meet several criteria, including ease of manufacturing, efficient gene transfer to target tissue, long-term gene expression to alleviate the disease, and most importantly safety in patients. The main rule of a gene therapeutic routine relies on the delivery of a corrected gene of interest in human cells such as Adenovirus vectors, Lentiviral vectors [41, 42], gamma-retroviral vectors are a reliable choice for use in gene therapy. However, Adenovirus vectors (AAV) have become popular for gene therapy due to their relative efficiency in gene delivery. AAV is currently the only known human DNA virus that is non-pathogenic and AAV-based vectors are classified as Risk Group 1 agents for all laboratory and animal studies. These vectors lack certain genes that are required for virus replication and therefore, have to be propagated in cell lines that complement the defect. Although such vectors are replication-defective, they should be handled at the same BSL as the parent adenovirus from which they are derived. The reason for this is that the virus stocks may be contaminated with replication-competent viruses, which are generated by rare spontaneous recombination events in the complementing cell line. The retroviral vectors, used in gene therapy and production of transgenic animals are risky as they can easily infect and propagate themselves in human cells. *Even defective retroviruses are infective and require a trained virologist* [43]. **The unpredictable consequences of hybridization and gene expression in host require strict precautions to fight any unwanted affect; for instance, a simple needle stick injury might turn out to be a precursor of a deadly disease.**

The gene therapy is under close scrutiny for potential concerns over biosafety. There are expert regulatory committees whose duty includes monitoring the pros and cons of any gene therapy study or pharmaceutical trial at all stages of experiment design and actual execution. **The biosafety of laboratory workers and patients in gene therapy laboratories involved in crucial task of manufacturing is the ethical and moral responsibility of the laboratory administration.** In countries like US, such laboratories come under law; agencies like National Institute of Health (NIH) and Food and Drug Administration (FDA) routinely update their guidelines for gene therapy.

### Transgenic and "Knock-Out" Animals

Any research on animals has to be performed in conformation to the norms issued from time to time. The countries under European Union follow the directive of European Union parliament, 2010 (Directive 2010/63/EU) [44], or annexure issued thereafter. The laboratories in US use the guidelines proposed by US Department of health and human services (BMBL, 2009) [45]. A transgenic animal is one that carries a foreign gene that has been **deliberately inserted** into its genome using **R-DNA methodology**. In addition to the gene itself, the DNA usually includes other sequences to enable it to be incorporated into the DNA of the host and to be expressed correctly by the cells of the host. These transgenic animals should be handled in the containment levels appropriate to the characteristics of the products of the foreign genes. Animals with targeted deletions of specific genes are known as "knock-out" animals. They do not generally present particular biological hazards. Examples of transgenic animals include animals expressing receptors for viruses normally unable to infect that species. If such animals escape from the laboratory and transmit the transgene to the wild animal population, an animal reservoir for that particular virus could theoretically be generated. This possibility has been discussed for poliovirus and is particularly relevant in the context of poliomyelitis eradication. Transgenic mice expressing the human poliovirus receptor generated in different laboratories were susceptible to poliovirus infection by various inoculation routes and the resulting disease was clinically and histopathologically similar to human poliomyelitis. However, the mouse model differs from humans in that alimentary tract replication of orally administered poliovirus is either inefficient or does not occur. Therefore, it is very unlikely that escape of such transgenic mice to the wild would result in the establishment of a new animal reservoir for poliovirus. However, this example indicates that for each new line of transgenic animal, detailed studies should be conducted to determine the routes by which the animals can be infected, the inoculum size required for infection and the extent of virus shedding by the infected animals. In addition, all measures should be taken to assure strict containment of receptor transgenic mice.

The risk associated with transgenic animal involves the following human health considerations.

1. Similarity of the recombinant organism to the wild-type organism regarding pathogenicity, transmission route to human, pathogenicity to humans (or to animals if appropriate).
2. Health considerations generally associated with the presence of non-viable organisms or with the products of rDNA processes.
3. Management of personnel exposure, including biological measures and physical and organizational measures. Any animal infected with retrovirus needs to be handled with extra care for scratches and bites.

**Transgenic Plants**

**Genetically modified transgenic plants have been created using R-DNA molecules.** Transgenic plants expressing genes that give tolerance to herbicides or resistance to insects are currently a matter of controversy in most parts of the world. *Transgenic plants expressing genes of animal or human origin should remain strictly contained within the facility.* Such transgenic plants should be handled at BSLs appropriate to the characteristics of the products of the expressed genes.

The risk associated with transgenic plant involves the following environmental and agricultural considerations.

1. Ecological traits relating to the donor and recipient environment.
2. Properties of environment where the engineered organisms are being applied.
3. Survival, multiplication and dissemination of the engineered organisms in the environment.
4. Interactions of engineered organism(s) with biological systems (target and non-target populations, stability, and routes of dissemination).
5. Potential environmental impacts such as effect on target and non-target organisms and ecosystems.

The principal investigator is responsible for implementing the necessary safety requirements in his/her laboratory. When creating or handling recombinant organisms, it is essential to perform a detailed risk assessment which must take into account the nature of the donor, the recipient organism and the environment. The **National Institute of Health (NIH),** which established guidelines for work with **Genetically Modified Organisms (GMOs)** help scientists classify their work at the appropriate **Biosafety Level (BSL)**. Risk assessment is thus a dynamic process and has to take into account new developments and the progress of science. It is the responsibility of the scientists involved in genetic engineering to keep up to date on these developments. For example, risk assessment is very important when creating GMOs expressing proteins with pharmacological activity, such as toxins. Some pharmacologically active proteins are only toxic when expressed at high levels. In this case, the risk assessment becomes very demanding and requires an estimation of the expected expression levels of the protein by a particular recombinant organism and the levels at which a given protein becomes toxic in an organism accidentally exposed to it. It is obvious that such organisms must be handled with caution.

What safety measures should be taken to control exposure to laboratory pathogens while at work?

In line with the agenda to minimize the hazards of occupational exposure to laboratory pathogens, an employer must employ an exposure control plan for the work station with emphasis on employee protection measures. The plan must shed light on the manner it proposes to employ fine union of engineering and work practice checks (Fig. **9**), ensuring the use of personal protective clothing and equipment, provide teaching and guidance, medical surveillance, vaccinations, and signs and labels, among other provisions. Engineering controls are the primary means of eliminating or minimizing employee exposure.

## How to Shield from Laboratory Infections?

It is imperative for a laboratory worker to familiarize himself about the kind of work being conducted in the laboratory, the biosafety levels involved, any laboratory specific protocols to be adopted, the availability of personal protective equipment besides getting acquainted with emergency medical and fire safety numbers. The three core areas of self defense in any laboratory include approach, personal protective equipment and organization.

## Attitude and Approach

The right attitude is treating all human or animal blood and body fluids/waste/tissue as infectious regardless of the perceived status of the source. '*Universal Safety Precautions*' should be adopted. Never

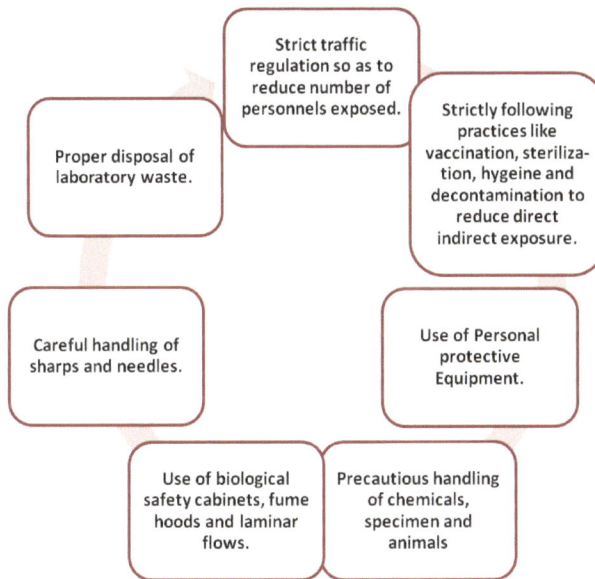

**Fig. (9).** Essential Strategic Areas for Biosafety.

should one try to break the recommended safety guidelines. This also means that certain engineering and work practice controls shall always be utilized in situations where exposure may occur.

**Right Personal Protective Equipment (PPE)**: It is undeniable that PPE should be used at all times to prevent skin or mucous membrane contact with bodily fluids. But, the user should always inspect PPE including lab coats, gloves, eye goggles, face shields, pocket mask, *etc.* for cracks, holes or other damage. PPE like gloves and gowns protect your skin and hands from coming into contact with blood/any infectious fluid/acid or alkali. Face Shield and eye protection do the same job to prevent blood/any infectious fluid/acid or alkali from entering the mucous membranes through eyes, nose or mouth.

**Housekeeping: Besides keeping the laboratory space organized and clutter free,** housekeeping also refers to methods of cleaning and decontaminating infected surfaces and the disposal of blood and body fluids. All decontaminations must include the use of an appropriate disinfecting solution, such as one-part bleach to ten parts water.

**Decontamination and sterilization:** All surfaces, tools, equipment and other objects that come in contact with blood or potentially infectious materials must be decontaminated and sterilized as soon as possible. Equipment and tools must be cleaned and decontaminated before servicing or being put back to use. **Detailed methods and standards for surface disinfection can be seen in EN 14885.** The methods of decontamination depend on concentration and type of target organism and duration of contact. They also depend on the nature of disinfectant used, water solubility, pH, mode of application [46]. Basically, there are two types of disinfectants available, surface disinfectant and airborne surface disinfectant. Airborne surface disinfectant is usually used during periodical cleaning or accidental spill.

The general method of decontamination should be accomplished by using:

1. A solution of 5.25% sodium hypochlorite (household bleach/Clorox) diluted between 1:10 and 1:100 with water. The standard recommendation is to use at least a quarter cup of bleach per one gallon of water.
2. Lysol/clorox or some other EPA-registered tuberculocidal disinfectant. Check the label of all disinfectants to make sure they meet this requirement.
3. If one is cleaning up a spill of blood, one can carefully cover the spill with paper towels or rags, then gently pour 10% solution of bleach over the towels or rags, and leave it for at least 10 minutes. This will help ensure that bloodborne pathogens are killed before one actually begins cleaning or wiping the material up. By covering the spill with paper towels or rags, you decrease the chances of causing a splash when you pour the bleach on it.
4. If you are decontaminating equipment or other objects (be it scalpels, microscope slides, broken glass, saw blades, tweezers, mechanical equipment upon which someone has been cut, first aid boxes, or whatever) you should

leave the disinfectant in place for at least 10 minutes before continuing the cleaning process.

5. Any material you use to clean up a spill of blood or potentially infectious materials must be decontaminated immediately, as well. This would include mops, sponges, re-usable gloves, buckets, pails, *etc.* Disposal of these materials is also very important (See biological waste disposal section of this chapter).

6. The decontamination procedure for any laboratory should be done conforming to the directives of prestigious agencies like European standards EN 14885 (Fig. **10**), or Occupational Safety and health administration's guidelines for Occupational exposure to bloodborne pathogens.

   European standards EN 14885 ensure active ingredients for sporicidal activity (NF EN 14347), mycobactericidal activity (NF EN 14348), virucidal activity (NF EN 14476 and NF EN 14675), fungicidal (EN 1650 and EN 1657+13624) and bactericidal activity (NF EN 1276 and EN 1656+EN 13727) are present in a disinfectant. European standards prefer other biocidal agents over formaldehyde.

   Alternatively, Environment Protection Agency (EPA) usually approves disinfectants based on their properties against common pathogens. The EPA approved products conform to the Occupational Safety and health administration's requirements for Occupational exposure to bloodborne pathogens. The EPA classifies various products into categories like sterilizers, tuberculocidal, virucidal *etc*. There are various other categories like products effective against medical waste or hepatitis which may be considered depending upon laboratory requirements.

7. Sanitization of cages in a BSL-2 laboratory requires washing them at 74°C for 6 minutes followed by a rinse of water at 82°C.This process has been found virucidal enough to clear adenovirus and viral vectors. However, simple washing or washing with a simple disinfectant failed to show any virucidal activity [47]. Traces of pathogens like mouse parvovirus, mouse hepatovirus, Helicobacter sp., Mycoplasma pulmonis, Sypacia obvelata and Myocopetes musculinus were found eliminated after a similar wash [48]. Recently, Hydrogen peroxide vapor has been shown to have bactericidal effect on cages [49].

**Universal Precautions or Rules to be followed for safety:** When you are working with blood or body fluids always follow '*Universal Precautions*'. Always wear personal protective equipment or PPE (Fig. **11**) in exposure situations. Vaccinations do not always ensure prevention from infection [32]. Therefore, one should never underscore the significance of personal protective equipment and safe laboratory practices.

a. Never ever use those PPE that has lost its ability to function as a barrier to bloodborne pathogens or harsh chemicals. Replace PPE that is torn or punctured

b. Always remove PPE before leaving the work area.

c. If you work in an area with routine exposure to blood or potentially infectious materials, the necessary PPE should be readily accessible. Contaminated gloves, clothing, PPE, or other materials should be placed in appropriately labeled bags or containers until it is disposed of, decontaminated, or laundered. It is important to find out where these bags or containers are located in your area before beginning your work.

d. Laboratory personnel should be educated and trained by the organization. Besides this, it is the duty of the personnel to familiarize the self with safety protocols especially in developing countries. Always remember to use universal precautions. If you find yourself in a situation where you have to come in contact with blood or other body fluids and you do not have any standard personal protective equipment handy, you can improvise as may happen in laboratories working on very little budget. Use a towel, plastic bag, or some other barrier to help avoid direct contact.

e. In case of accidental needle prick injury of a known pathogen, laboratory supervisor and health clinics should be immediately informed. This step reduces the severity of infection and spread of infection. **Contract tracing** is required if colleagues get in touch of any infected fluid/exodus during rescue.

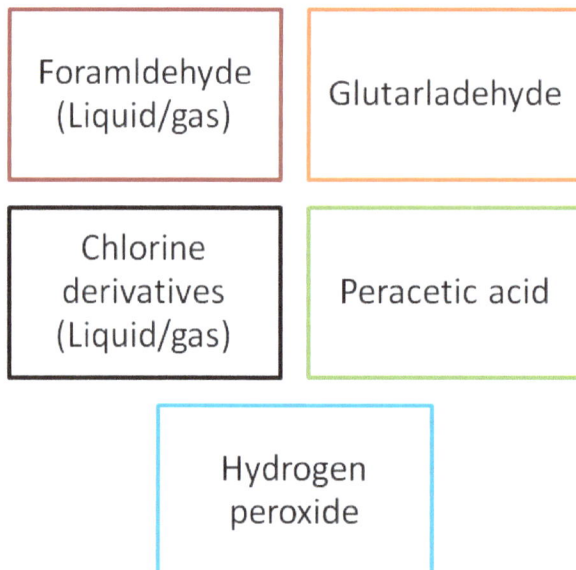

**Fig. (10).** Some commonly used biocides for disinfection.

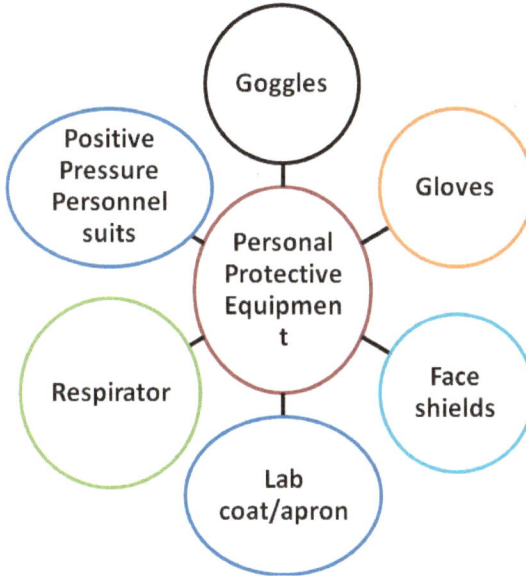

**Fig. (11).** Personal Protective Equipment.

## Personal Protective Equipment (PPE)

**Gloves:** Suitable gloves can be chosen from a wide array of available choices like latex, nitrile, rubber, or other water/chemical impervious materials as discussed in detail earlier in the chapter according to the nature of work and individual sensitivity of the researcher. With the increasing frequency of latex allergies nitrile or neoprene gloves are recommended. The gloves to be used in BSL-3 laboratory according to the EN 374 European standard, should have a 'microorganism' pictogram indicating that the gloves conform to at least performance level 2 for penetration test. If glove material is thin or flimsy, double gloving can provide an additional layer of protection. It is advised to wear double layer of gloves to avoid direct touch of toxin to bare skin. Also, if you know you have cuts or sores on your hands, you should cover those with a bandage or similar protection as an additional precaution before donning your gloves. You should always inspect your gloves for tears or punctures before putting them on. *If a glove is damaged, do not use it.* When taking contaminated gloves off, do so carefully. Make sure you don't touch the outside of the gloves with any bare skin, and be sure to dispose them in a proper container so that no one else comes in contact with them, either. Moreover, gloves should be the last PPE item to be worn.

**Lab. Coats/Aprons:** The committee of European standards routinely issues directives on the category of the kind of material for cloth of laboratory personnel depending on the nature work (Fig. **12**). Aprons may be worn to protect your clothing and to keep blood or other contaminated fluids from soaking through your skin. Normal clothing that becomes contaminated with blood should be removed as soon as possible because fluids can seep through the cloth to come into direct contact with skin. Contaminated laundry should be handled as little as possible, and it should be placed in an appropriately labeled bag or container until it is decontaminated, disposed of, or laundered.

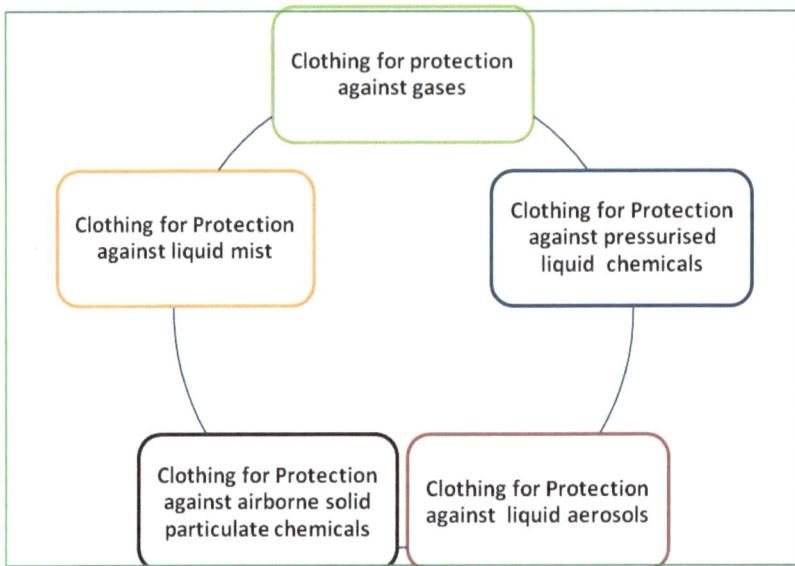

**Fig. (12).** Various categories of clothing material depending on probability of exposure.

**Respirators:** Concentration of agent, anticipated bioaerosol size and microorganisms are criteria for selecting a respirator. N95 mask is used for routine work in BSL 1 and 2 laboratories. BSL 3 facilities use powered purifying respirator which may or may not be valved. These respirators are also called as positive pressure masks. They have various categories of filters depending on particle size in compliance with European Norms 147 and 149. The positive pressure masks often come with eye protection.

**Eye protection:** If at any time there is a risk of splashing or vaporization of contaminated fluids eye protection should be used to protect one's eyes. Again, bloodborne pathogens can be transmitted through the thin membranes of the eyes so it is important to protect them. Splashing could occur while cleaning up a spill, during laboratory procedures, or while providing first aid or medical assistance.

**Face Shields:** Face shields may be worn in addition to goggles to provide additional face protection. A face shield will protect against splashes to the nose and mouth.

**Hygiene Practices:** Handwashing is one of the most crucial and easiest practices to prevent transmission of bloodborne pathogens. Hands or other exposed skin should be thoroughly washed as soon as possible following an exposure incident. If possible, use soft antibacterial soap. Avoid harsh, abrasive soaps, as these may open fragile scabs or other sores. Hands should also be washed immediately after removal of gloves or other personal protective equipment.

One should know the location of the nearest hand washing facilities. Laboratory sinks, public restrooms, and so forth may be used for hand washing if they are normally supplied with soap. If one is working in an area without access to such facilities, one may use an antiseptic cleanser in conjunction with clean cloth/paper towels or antiseptic towelettes. If these alternative methods are used, hands should be washed with soap and running water as soon as possible.

**What to do if one is exposed to infectious material?** Despite one's best efforts, there is a possibility that one and co-workers may be exposed to infectious tissue like blood or body fluids or acids or alkalis during an experimental or routine procedure (Fig. **13**). Depending on the probability of exposure there are three risk categories of people - low risk, medium risk and high risk. Protect yourself immediately and after that treat the victim. If you have an exposure, follow these steps:

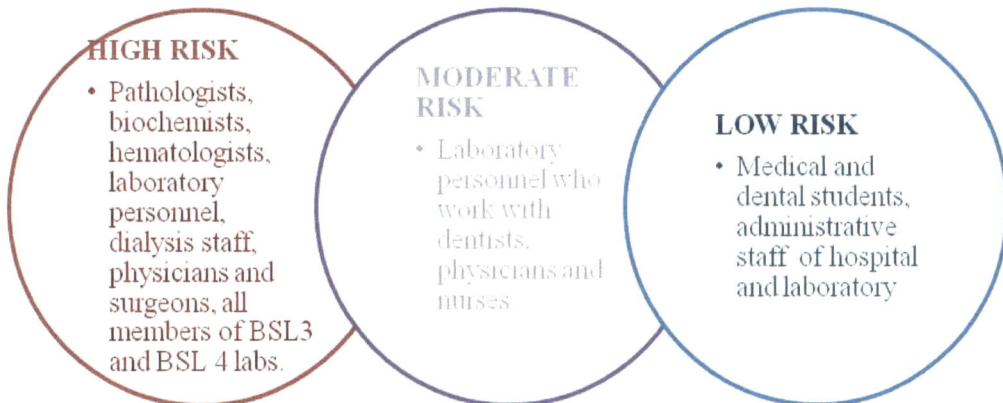

**Fig. (13).** The risk categories depending on the probability of exposure.

Wash the exposed area thoroughly with soap and running water. Vigorously scrub all areas for 30 seconds. It is the abrasive action of scrubbing that removes contaminates from the skin. If you have an open wound, squeeze gently to make it bleed, then wash with soap and water. If possible use non-abrasive, antibacterial soap. These days, alcohol based hand rubs are used.

1. If blood is splashed in the eye or mucous membrane, flush the affected area with running water for at least 15 minutes.
2. Report the exposure to your supervisor as soon as possible. Seek emergency medical treatment following an exposure incident.

## Biological Waste Disposal

Large amount of biological waste is generated in research, teaching and clinical laboratories. Animal carcasses, infectious excreta & bedding, blood & blood products, pathological waste, parasites, recombinant products, allergens, cultures of human and animal cells, live and attenuated vaccines all are potential bio-hazardous agents. These agents may contain, infected clinical specimens, tissue from experimental animals, plant viruses, bacteria and fungi, toxins *etc.* Biological wastes require proper disposal; otherwise, it may turn out to be a source of contamination culminating in a potential health hazard with infectious organisms or agents. These bio-hazardous agents might be capable of self-replication or may serve as breeding ground for other infectious biological organisms or may release harmful toxic compounds.

**Cultures** for disposal of such wastes like, biologically-cultured stocks and petri dishes, surgical wraps, culture tubes, human or animal blood or tissues, blood vials, absorbent material, personal protective equipment and pipette tips *etc.* The lab personnel should sterilize or disinfect waste materials associated with viral, bacterial or other agents infectious to humans by *autoclave or chemical treatment equivalent to 1:10 bleach solution.* **Do not autoclave containers or other receptacles containing bleach.** The combination of bleach and residual cotton and oil (improperly cleaned autoclaves) may result in an explosive combustion within the autoclave. All bio-hazardous wastes, except sharps should directly be put into medical waste boxes provided. Laboratory personnel must apply an adhesive-backed label completed with generator information to each bag or container (such as autoclaved bags or filled sharps containers) before placing garbage into the medical waste box.

**Research animal waste** The contaminated carcasses, blood or blood products, pathological waste, body parts and bedding of animals *etc.* that were intentionally exposed to infectious agents during research or testing are categorized under **Research animal waste**. Animal bedding waste and all animal carcasses that have been exposed to biosafety level 2 agents need to be autoclaved prior to disposal or, if an autoclave is not available in the animal facility it should be packaged as infectious waste in cardboard fiber drums or boxes by Laboratory Animal Resources (LAR) staff. Infectious waste containers are picked up by building services and transported to a weather-protected shelter for holding until they are picked up by the institution's infectious waste vendor, for incineration. Spills from containers of animal bedding labeled as infectious waste are to be cleaned up by LAR staff. Animal bedding that has not been labeled as infectious is bagged and collected for disposal by LAR staff. Any spill of non-infectious bedding when loading the truck is cleaned up by the building services trash crew. Washing the cages at 74°C for 6 minutes followed by a rinse of water at 82°C is an approved method of sterilization of cages. This process has been shown to be virucidal [47], bactericidal [48].

Bags are filled only to a specified intensity and weight that will allow for effective tying of the bag by animal facility staff. For example, several partially-filled bags should be tied and placed in the gray carts rather than one or two full bags. This will help in preventing repetitive motion injury to staff and prevents bags from being ripped open while being handled. The carts are maintained clean in sanitary condition by the animal facility staff.

In each animal facility, freezers are provided for storage of carcasses that have been bagged and sealed. Freezers are cleaned and defrosted by animal laboratory personnel to keep them in a sanitary condition.

**Isolation Waste:** Biological waste and discarded material contaminated with body fluids from humans or animals which are isolated because they are known to be infected with a highly communicable disease (biosafety level 4 agent). HIV-containing cell or tissue cultures, organ cultures and HIV- or HBV-containing culture medium or other solutions, and blood, organs, or other tissues from experimental animals infected with HIV or HBV. "Look-alike" infectious waste is defined as laboratory materials that can be used to contain, transfer or mix infectious agents but has been used with non-infectious agents. For example, disposable micropipette tips may have transferred sterile water or broth, but an identical tip in the same laboratory may have transferred an infectious agent in the trash you could not distinguish between them. These 'look-alike' materials will be handled as infectious waste if the facility routinely generates infectious or potentially infectious biological waste or is engaged in a temporary project that generates infectious or potentially infectious biological waste.

**Biological *Versus* Chemical Waste:** Biological and chemical waste must be managed separately. In order to clarify how these various wastes are to be handled in laboratories using biological materials, the waste classification chart can be created and pasted in the laboratory. Follow the formula below to determine the waste stream.

1. Biological + Radiation = Radiation Waste
2. Biological + Hazardous Chemical = Chemical Waste

The most common example is Agarose gel contaminated with Ethidium Bromide or heavy metals (*e.g.,* arsenic, chromium). This kind of material should always be treated as chemical waste. When laboratory produces both biological and chemical waste then biological waste should be treated first. Once the biological agents have been deactivated by either autoclave or chemical disinfection, the remaining chemical waste should be submitted to the proper authority. If the laboratories produce large amount of chemical waste, then they should construct weather resistant sealed pits. Although detailed account of what can't go down the drain is beyond the scope of the book, (Fig. **14**) briefly outlines a generalized guideline. Given below are some examples of chemicals which should be treated first before going to drain.

| | | |
|---|---|---|
| Oil/Grease/paint/solids/ash | Radioactive waste | Chemical waste based on corrosive pH levels between pH 2 and 5 or $\leq 2$ or $\geq 12$ |
| Untreated biohazardoius waste | Dilute solutions of inorganic salts like Arsenic, Barium, Cadmium, Mercury, Lead, Selenium, Silver | Very high temperature 150° F Liquids or explosives or flammable liquids. |
| Alcohols (only 24% ethnol is allowed) | Formalin (only solutions having 2.9% formaldehyde is allowed) | Hydrogen peroxide (only concentrations $\leq 8$) |
| Mercaptans, Nitro & Halogenated compounds (like chloroform) | Any gel forming water soluble chemicals. | Substances with low boiling points below 50 °F. |

Fig. (**14**). What can't go down the drain?

- If solution has Cyanide, it should be converted to carbonate using excess sodium hypochlorite.
- If solution has Zinc sulphide, it can be precipitated as Zinc sulphate, rest of the solution can be drained.
- If solution has Chromium VI it should be reduced to Chromium III.
- If one has chlorinated and non-chlorinated solvent carrying wastes, then keep them separately.
- *If the chemical nature of waste is uncertain deal it as chemical hazardous waste until a determination can be made. Consult peers.*
- *Paste this information near laboratory sink.*

**Other Wastes:** Certain wastes that are generated in these facilities that are not contaminated with biological agents or materials are not treated as bio-hazardous and may be discarded in the regular trash container, with recyclables, or into other specially designated waste containers. These include such items as recyclable and non-recyclable wastes like glass, gloves, unused plates.

**Liquid Waste:** Liquid biological waste should be collected in containers for **autoclaving or chemical disinfection**. Autoclaved or chemically disinfected liquid wastes can be poured down the drain (sanitary sewer) under running water. The sanitary sewer should have been designed for the disposal of certain liquid wastes. Use of the sanitary sewer reduces the chance for leaks or spills during transport and reduces disposal costs. Human or animal blood and body fluids do not need to be disinfected before being poured down the drain but some institutions are disinfecting blood before pouring carefully down the drain. The sink should be rinsed well and disinfected if necessary after the disposal procedure.

**Solid Waste:** Solid biological waste, including solidified agarose gels, should be collected in appropriate bio-hazardous waste autoclave bags. Once the waste has been autoclaved or chemically disinfected, the autoclave bags should be taped or tied shut and placed inside of the cardboard box provided by the institute.

**Radioactive Waste**: Radioactive wastes are wastes that contain radioactive material. The Radiation Safety Section is responsible for the radioactive waste.

1. All the radioactive waste should be kept separately and not in regular containers.
2. Any radioactive animal tissue, carcass, dry waste, infectious waste, sharps, gel *etc.* Should be kept in separate bags filling only up to ¾ of the bag. Line it with enough absorbent material to prevent any leakage.
3. Liquid radioactive waste should always be stored within a secondary container

only up to the indicated mark.

4. Attach hazardous/infectious waste tag listing all contents, if it has any other waste along with radioactive waste.
5. NEVER use any formula or abbreviation on tags. Always write in full.
6. All radioactive wastes should be separated by isotopes specially Iodine. Iodine waste has separate requirements; therefore, it should be stored separately.

**Transport:** Transfer of any biological material can turn out to be an occupational (biological) hazard. If researchers are receiving or sending any material to a distant laboratory or to a laboratory within the institute, they must get familiar with transportation protocols like WHO (2012) and adhere to uniform code of conduct to avoid any mishap to self or recipient. The United Nations committee of experts on the transport of Dangerous Goods **(UNCETDG)** issues protocol to transport any infectious substance. It carries instructions to packing lest any research personnel unknowingly open it and get exposed. Training and education in packing and shipping hazardous laboratory material is necessary for all laboratory staff [49, 50]. All the category A substances require triple layer packing. There are specific codes meant for packing which are essential to be mentioned on the label so that the person opening the material might take relevant precautions *e.g.,* Code UN2814 indicates the material is life threatening to both humans and animals, while code UN 2900 indicates the material is life threatening to animals.

**Training** all employees who handle biological waste should be trained regarding the proper segregation, handling, packaging, labeling, storage, and treatment of biological wastes. Refresher training is required annually. One should not use any laboratory equipment or procedure without adequate training.

## CONCLUSION

As biotechnology and synthetic biology take center stage, biological risks and laboratory acquired infections are inevitable. Biosecurity and biosafety have emerged as major areas of concern. Institutional biosafety committees are the first checkpoints to review any possible biological hazards in research organizations. Environmental health and safety department and occupational health departments in respective countries foresee release of any toxic product or harmful pathogen from the controlled laboratory environment which might affect laboratory personnel, general public and environment. These organization also provide help to the institutions with regard to fire safety, biological safety, chemical safety, radiological safety *etc.* All institutions must have their internal safety guidelines depending on niche requirement which the laboratory personnel should follow strictly. Appropriate training, facilities, apparatus, techniques reduce the risk of laboratory acquired infection substantially. Despite advances in laboratory design technology, available tools, knowledge regarding biosafety and adequate training in internationally recognized safe practices laboratory acquired infections do occur [51]. Techniques like Pulse Field Gel Electrophoresis (PFGE), Serotyping and whole genome sequencing might replace traditional diagnostic methods to identify the strain and hence the management of the ailment.

The laboratories working on GMO or biosafety level 3/4 turn out to be very expensive. The running cost of laboratory is very high as the labs need to get yearly certification of their HEPA filter, HVAC, autoclaves, biosafety cabinets *etc.* This means the laboratories require adequate funding. Therefore, it is imperative that institutional leadership emerges from within the scientific community so that it deeply understands workplace issues.

## CONSENT FOR PUBLICATION

Not applicable.

## ACKNOWLEDGEMENTS

Declared none

## CONFLICT OF INTEREST

The authors confirm that this contents of this chapter have no conflict of interest.

## REFERENCES

[1]   Sewell DL. Laboratory-associated infections and biosafety. Clin Microbiol Rev 1995; 8(3): 389-405.
      [http://dx.doi.org/10.1128/CMR.8.3.389] [PMID: 7553572]

[2]   Siengsanan-Lamont J, Blacksell SD. A Review of Laboratory-Acquired Infections in the Asia-Pacific: Understanding Risk and the Need for Improved Biosafety for Veterinary and Zoonotic Diseases. Trop Med Infect Dis 2018; 3(2): E36.
      [http://dx.doi.org/10.3390/tropicalmed3020036] [PMID: 30274433]

[3]   Quddus M, Jehan M, Ali NH. Hepatitis-b vaccination status and knowledge, attitude and practice of high risk health care worker about body substance isolation. J Ayub Med Coll Abbottabad 2015; 27(3): 664-8.
      [PMID: 26721035]

[4]   Biosafety in the Laboratory: Prudent Practices for Handling and Disposal of Infectious Materials. Washington (DC): National Academies Press 1989; pp. 1-216.

[5]   Keith Furr A. CRC Handbook of Laboratory Safety. 5$^{th}$ ed. United States: CRC Press 2000; pp. 1-808.
      [http://dx.doi.org/10.1201/9781420038460]

[6]   Biological Risk Assessment," in Biosafety in Microbiological and Biomedical Laboratories. 5th ed. Washington, DC: U.S. Government Printing Office 2009; pp. 10-3.

[7]   Whistler T, Kaewpan A, Blacksell SD. A Biological Safety Cabinet Certification Program: Experiences in Southeast Asia. Appl Biosaf 2016; 21(3): 121-7.
      [http://dx.doi.org/10.1177/1535676016661769] [PMID: 27721674]

[8]     Homer LC, Alderman TS, Blair HA, *et al.* Guidelines for biosafety training programs for workers
        assigned to BSL-3 research laboratories. Biosecur Bioterror 2013; 11(1): 10-9.
        [http://dx.doi.org/10.1089/bsp.2012.0038] [PMID: 23477631]

[9]     Rusnak JM, Kortepeter MG, Hawley RJ, Anderson AO, Boudreau E, Eitzen E. Risk of occupationally
        acquired illnesses from biological threat agents in unvaccinated laboratory workers. Biosecur Bioterror
        2004; 2(4): 281-93.
        [http://dx.doi.org/10.1089/bsp.2004.2.281] [PMID: 15650438]

[10]    Lee C, Jang EJ, Kwon D, Choi H, Park JW, Bae GR. Laboratory-acquired dengue virus infection by
        needlestick injury: a case report, South Korea, 2014. Ann Occup Environ Med 2016; 28: 16.
        [http://dx.doi.org/10.1186/s40557-016-0104-5] [PMID: 27057314]

[11]    Wallach JC, Giambartolomei GH, Baldi PC, Fossati CA. Human infection with M- strain of Brucella
        canis. Emerg Infect Dis 2004; 10(1): 146-8.
        [http://dx.doi.org/10.3201/eid1001.020622] [PMID: 15078613]

[12]    Lowe CF, Showler AJ, Perera S, *et al.* Hospital-associated transmission of Brucella melitensis outside
        the laboratory. Emerg Infect Dis 2015; 21(1): 150-2.
        [http://dx.doi.org/10.3201/eid2101.141247] [PMID: 25531198]

[13]    Fiori PL, Mastrandrea S, Rappelli P, Cappuccinelli P. Brucella abortus infection acquired in
        microbiology laboratories. J Clin Microbiol 2000; 38(5): 2005-6.
        [PMID: 10790142]

[14]    Wever PC, Hodges AJ. The First World War years of Sydney Domville Rowland: an early case of
        possible laboratory-acquired meningococcal disease. J R Army Med Corps 2016; 162(4): 310-5.
        [http://dx.doi.org/10.1136/jramc-2016-000634] [PMID: 27084843]

[15]    Sheets CD, Harriman K, Zipprich J, *et al.* Fatal meningococcal disease in a laboratory worker-
        -California, 2012. MMWR Morb Mortal Wkly Rep 2014; 63(35): 770-2.
        [PMID: 25188495]

[16]    Hong E, Terrade A, Taha MK. Immunogenicity and safety among laboratory workers vaccinated with
        Bexsero® vaccine. Hum Vaccin Immunother 2017; 13(3): 645-8.
        [http://dx.doi.org/10.1080/21645515.2016.1241358] [PMID: 27808594]

[17]    Gaspar MP, Landes G, Safavi F, Osterman AL. Accidental injection of freund complete adjuvant with
        mycobacterium tuberculosis. J Hand Surg Am 2018; 43(9): 873.e1-4.
        [http://dx.doi.org/10.1016/j.jhsa.2018.02.008] [PMID: 29526530]

[18]    van Soolingen D, Wisselink HJ, Lumb R, Anthony R, van der Zanden A, Gilpin C. Practical biosafety
        in the tuberculosis laboratory: containment at the source is what truly counts. Int J Tuberc Lung Dis
        2014; 18(8): 885-9.
        [http://dx.doi.org/10.5588/ijtld.13.0629] [PMID: 25199000]

[19]    Ridzon R, Kenyon T, Luskin-Hawk R, Schultz C, Valway S, Onorato IM. Nosocomial transmission of
        human immunodeficiency virus and subsequent transmission of multidrug-resistant tuberculosis in a
        healthcare worker. nfect Control Hosp Epidemiol 1997; 18(6): 422-3.

[20]    Shapiro DS, Schwartz DR. Exposure of laboratory workers to Francisella tularensis despite a
        bioterrorism procedure. J Clin Microbiol 2002; 40(6): 2278-81.
        [http://dx.doi.org/10.1128/JCM.40.6.2278-2281.2002] [PMID: 12037110]

[21]    Centers for disease control and prevention (cdc).. anthrax in a laboratoryworker--texas, 2002. mmwr
        morb mortal wkly rep 2002; 51(13): 279-81.

[22]    Alexander DC, Fitzgerald SF, DePaulo R, *et al.* Laboratory-acquired infection with salmonella
        enterica serovar typhimurium exposed by whole-genome sequencing. J Clin Microbiol 2016; 54(1):
        190-3.
        [http://dx.doi.org/10.1128/JCM.02720-15] [PMID: 26511736]

[23]   Mughini-Gras L, Schaapveld M, Kramers J, *et al.* Increased colon cancer risk after severe Salmonella infection. PLoS One 2018; 13(1): e0189721.
[http://dx.doi.org/10.1371/journal.pone.0189721]

[24]   Takada S, Andou T, Yamaguchi K, Tokuda Y. A febrile microbiologist. BMJ Case Rep 2016; 2016: bcr2016216229.
[http://dx.doi.org/10.1136/bcr-2016-216229] [PMID: 27298297]

[25]   Smith AM, Smouse SL, Tau NP, *et al.* Laboratory-acquired infections of Salmonella enterica serotype Typhi in South Africa: phenotypic and genotypic analysis of isolates. BMC Infect Dis 2017; 17(1): 656.
[http://dx.doi.org/10.1186/s12879-017-2757-2] [PMID: 28962627]

[26]   Yuet-Meng Cheong, Tikki Pang. A probable case of laboratory-acquired infection with salmonella typhi: Evidence from phage typing, antibiograms, and analysis by pulsed-field gel electrophoresis. International Journal of Infectious DiseasesVolume 1996; 1(2): 95-7.
[http://dx.doi.org/10.1016/S1201-9712(96)90061-2]

[27]   L A. Mermel, S L. Josephson, J Dempsey, S Parenteau, C Perry, N Magill. Leonard A.MermelStephen L.JosephsonJaneDempseyStephenParenteauChristopherPerryNancyMagillOutbreak of Shigella sonnei in a clinical microbiology laboratory. J Clin Micro 1997; 35(12): 3163-5.

[28]   Blacksell SD, Robinson MT, Newton PN, Day NPJ. Laboratory-acquired scrub typhus and murine typhus infections: The argument for risk-based approach to biosafety requirements for Orientia tsutsugamushi and Rickettsia typhi laboratory activities. Clin Infect Dis 2018. Epub ahead of print
[http://dx.doi.org/10.1093/cid/ciy675] [PMID: 30107504]

[29]   Ohnishi K. Needle-stick dengue virus infection in a health-care worker at a Japanese hospital. J Occup Health 2015; 57(5): 482-3.
[http://dx.doi.org/10.1539/joh.14-0224-CS] [PMID: 26084918]

[30]   Khabour OF, Al Ali KH, Mahallawi WH. Occupational infection and needle stick injury among clinical laboratory workers in Al-Madinah city, Saudi Arabia. J Occup Med Toxicol 2018 May 21; 13: 15.

[31]   Motlagh ZM, Mokhtari A, Mahzounieh M. Genomic identification of human vaccinia virus keratoconjunctivitis and its importance as a laboratory-acquired infection. Indian J Ophthalmol 2016; 64(11): 806-12.
[http://dx.doi.org/10.4103/0301-4738.195592] [PMID: 27958202]

[32]   Hsu CH, Farland J, Winters T, *et al.* Laboratory-acquired vaccinia virus infection in a recently immunized person--Massachusetts, 2013. MMWR Morb Mortal Wkly Rep 2015; 64(16): 435-8.
[PMID: 25928468]

[33]   Venter M, Burt FJ, Blumberg L, Fickl H, Paweska J, Swanepoel R. Cytokine induction after laboratory-acquired West Nile virus infection. N Engl J Med 2009; 360(12): 1260-2.
[http://dx.doi.org/10.1056/NEJMc0808647] [PMID: 19297584]

[34]   Shi X, McCaughey C, Elliott RM. Genetic characterisation of a Hantavirus isolated from a laboratory-acquired infection. J Med Virol 2003; 71(1): 105-9.
[http://dx.doi.org/10.1002/jmv.10446] [PMID: 12858415]

[35]   Li Z, Li J, Zhang Y, *et al.* Aerosolized avian influenza virus by laboratory manipulations. Virol J 2012; 9: 146.
[http://dx.doi.org/10.1186/1743-422X-9-146] [PMID: 22866888]

[36]   Herwaldt BL. Laboratory-acquired parasitic infections from accidental exposures. Clin Microbiol Rev 2001; 14(4): 659-88.
[http://dx.doi.org/10.1128/CMR.14.3.659-688.2001] [PMID: 11585780]

[37]   Emery DW. Big changes coming to biosafety oversight of clinical gene transfer. Mol Ther 2014; 22(8): 1402.

[http://dx.doi.org/10.1038/mt.2014.122] [PMID: 25082087]

[38]   Chan CT, Lee JW, Cameron DE, Bashor CJ, Collins JJ. 'Deadman' and 'Passcode' microbial kill switches for bacterial containment. Nat Chem Biol 2016; 12(2): 82-6.
[http://dx.doi.org/10.1038/nchembio.1979] [PMID: 26641934]

[39]   Jia B, Qi H, Li BZ, *et al.* Orthogonal ribosome biofirewall. ACS Synth Biol 2017; 6(11): 2108-17.
[http://dx.doi.org/10.1021/acssynbio.7b00148] [PMID: 28783349]

[40]   Yao J, Fan Y, Li Y, Huang L. Strategies on the nuclear-targeted delivery of genes. J Drug Target 2013; 21(10): 926-39.
[http://dx.doi.org/10.3109/1061186X.2013.830310] [PMID: 23964565]

[41]   Pauwels K, Gijsbers R, Toelen J, *et al.* State-of-the-art lentiviral vectors for research use: risk assessment and biosafety recommendations. Curr Gene Ther 2009; 9(6): 459-74.
[http://dx.doi.org/10.2174/156652309790031120] [PMID: 20021330]

[42]   Howard J, Murashov V, Schulte P. Synthetic biology and occupational risk. J Occup Environ Hyg 2017; 14(3): 224-36.
[http://dx.doi.org/10.1080/15459624.2016.1237031] [PMID: 27754800]

[43]   Le Duc JW, Anderson K, Bloom ME, *et al.* Framework for leadership and training of Biosafety Level 4 laboratory workers. Emerg Infect Dis 2008; 14(11): 1685-8.
[http://dx.doi.org/10.3201/eid1411.080741] [PMID: 18976549]

[44]   Le Duc JW, Anderson K, Bloom ME, *et al.* Framework for leadership and training of Biosafety Level 4 laboratory workers. Emerg Infect Dis 2008; 14(11): 1685-8.
[http://dx.doi.org/10.3201/eid1411.080741] [PMID: 18976549]

[45]   Biosafety in Microbiological and Biomedical Laboratories 2009. http://www.cdc.gov/biosafety/publications/bmbl5/BMBL.pdf

[46]   Pastorino B, de Lamballerie X, Charrel R. Biosafety and biosecurity in european containment level 3 laboratories: Focus on french recent progress and essential requirements. Front Public Health 2017; 5: 121.
[http://dx.doi.org/10.3389/fpubh.2017.00121] [PMID: 28620600]

[47]   Porter JD, Lyons RM. Virucidal effects of rodent cage-cleaning practices on the viability of adenovirus vectors. Contemp Top Lab Anim Sci 2002; 41(5): 43-6.
[PMID: 12213048]

[48]   Compton SR, Macy JD. Effect of cage-wash temperature on the removal of infectious agents from caging and the detection of infectious agents on the filters of animal bedding-disposal cabinets by PCR analysis. J Am Assoc Lab Anim Sci 2015; 54(6): 745-55.
[PMID: 26632784]

[49]   Benga L, Benten WPM, Engelhardt E, Gougoula C, Schulze-Röbbecke R, Sager M. Survival of bacteria of laboratory animal origin on cage bedding and inactivation by hydrogen peroxide vapour. Lab Anim 2017; 51(4): 412-21.
[http://dx.doi.org/10.1177/0023677216675386] [PMID: 27932683]

[50]   World Health Organization (WHO). Guidance on Regulations for the Transport of Infectious Substances 2013-2014. Geneva 2012. WHO/HSE/GCR/2012.12.

[51]   Coelho AC, García Díez J. Biological risks and laboratory-acquired infections: A reality that cannot be ignored in health biotechnology. Front Bioeng Biotechnol 2015; 3: 56.
[http://dx.doi.org/10.3389/fbioe.2015.00056] [PMID: 25973418]

# CHAPTER 6

# Stress and Compromised Mental Health as The New Age Occupational Hazard

Farhana Zahir[*]

*Prism educational Society, Aligarh, U.P., India*

**Abstract:** Stress is a 21st century biproduct of globalization coupled with industrialization. WHO recognizes stress as one of the biggest challenges of our time. Two theoretical models are accepted to study stressful psychosocial work environment Job-Demand-Control (JDC) and Effort Reward Imbalance (ERI) or Organizational Justice (OJ) model. The work stressors like accumulating anxiety, insomnia or excessive sleepiness and depression coupled with lack of job satisfaction, diminished social life due to work pressure might lead to burn out occasionally leading to suicidal tendencies among workers. Shift work and migration are other major contributors to stress. A growing body of research underlines the significance of sleep for regeneration as good quality of sleep improves attention, focus and ameliorates stress. Sleep-wake cycle is regulated through neurons in hypothalamus as clock genes and Melatonin synchronize circadian rhythm which in turn influences emotion, behavior and cognition. Stress is a precursor of many disorders. Stress negatively stimulates Hypothalamic-Pituitary-adrenal axis and Autonomic Nervous System while circadian rhythm collapses during ageing. Allostatic adjustments are undertaken to maintain Homeostasis to prevent disease. The dysregulation of Allostatsis end in tertiary outcomes like cancer, depression, stroke, obesity, diabetes, Alzheimer's disease. Organizations are encouraged now-a-days by researchers to educate workers regarding sleep as a component of workers' health. Proper sleep is like basic practice of sanitation and hygiene which if properly undertaken helps avert a number of health related issues.

**Keywords:** Stress, anxiety, depression, behaviour, work stressor's, economic health, sleep, sleep-wake cycle, circadian rhythm, regeneration, Homeostasis, Allostatsis, Alzheimer's disease, migration, burn out, shift work, melatonin, Suprachiasmatic Nucleus (SCN).

## INTRODUCTION

Poor Mental health was earlier synonymous with problems related to mental retardation. Though, the scenario has changed. There is growing awareness of

---
[*] **Corresponding author Farhana Zahir:** Prism educational Society, Aligarh, U.P., India; Tel: +91 9760986931/+91 798386098; Email: farhanazahir@gmail.com

workers' mental health issues. The world has shrunk to be a smaller place and life is viewed as a race, every single professional wants to win. *Multitasking* has become a necessity; a range of gadgets is available to save time. Time has earned a new sobriquet "*deadline*". The pressure to perform and deliver gradually reaches medical proportions. *World Health organization* accepts stress to be a major health challenge for employers worldwide for the 21$^{st}$ century leading to absenteeism, early retirements, job terminations, low productivity, accidents and a series of health disorders. *Stress* is a byproduct of globalization coupled with industrialization. Stress is a 21$^{st}$ century phenomenon with roots in shrinking time and expansion of industrialization in a global village. European Survey of Enterprises on New and emerging risk (ESENER) in the year 2010 identified workrelated stress as the second biggest threat to occupational welfare [1].

## How the Organization is Affected by the Worker who is under Stress?

The worker under stress is unable to perform. The quality and quantity of his work suffer; this directly affects the economic health and prestige of the organization (Fig. **1**). The dissatisfied worker may take an early retirement. Moreover, mentally ill worker is prone to accidents keeping his own and fellow workers' safety at risk. A healthy mind and body means a productive worker and a successful organization. Therefore, a lot of research is now-a-days conducted to identify *work stressors* which perturb the employee. Workers are an asset of any establishment. Any good organization understands the value of a dedicated, skilled and loyal worker.

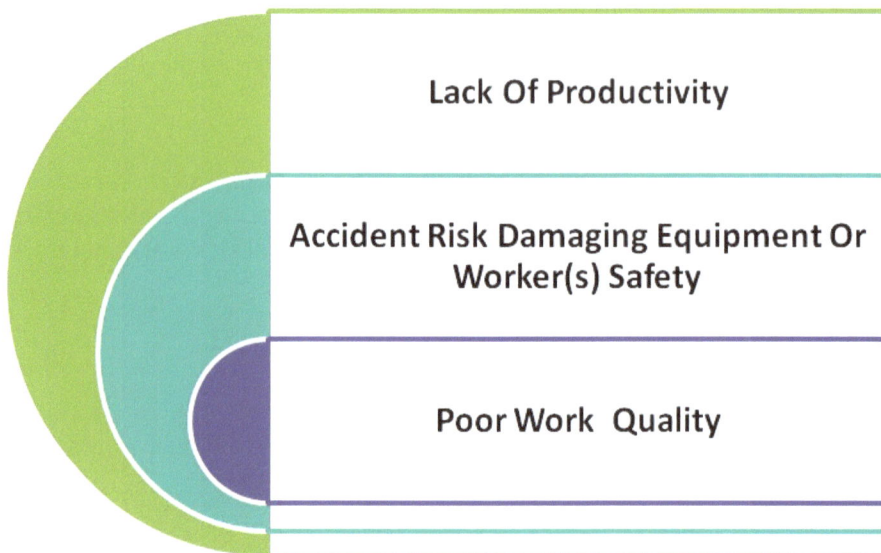

**Lack Of Productivity**

**Accident Risk Damaging Equipment Or Worker(s) Safety**

**Poor Work Quality**

**Fig. (1).** The effect of worker stress on economic health of the company.

Workplace stress has a constantly evolving and complex dynamics. It begins with work overload along with lack of reward. The accumulating anxiety, insomnia or excessive sleepiness and depression coupled with lack of job satisfaction, diminished social life due to work pressure might lead to burn out occasionally leading to suicidal tendencies among workers.

Two theoretical models are accepted to study stressful psychosocial work environment *Job-Demand-Control* (**JDC**) and *Effort Reward Imbalance* (**ERI**). **Job-Demand-Control (JDC) model** given by Robert Karasek in 1979 says that **control** (authority, decision making, confidentiality) of worker at workplace determines his workplace stress. **Job demands** include time required, interruption rate, deadline pressure, amount of work, slowest step is rate limiting, required degree of attention. Passive, active, low strain and high strain are four kinds of jobs according to **JDC model**. A number of studies were undertaken to understand the interaction between job demands (work overload/emotional demands) and resources (autonomy, social support and learning opportunities) which subsequently lead to worker burn out [2]. A cross sectional study conducted on critical care nurses in Spain revealed age, marital status, smoking habits as contributory factors leading to burn out syndrome [3]. The ever increasing job demands lead to drain in energy reserves culminating in emotional and physical exhaustion. **Effort reward Imbalance (ERI) model** was given by Siegrist in 1986. According to **ERI Model** if high efforts are rewarded with low awards, it will lead to unnecessary strain on health of the worker. Lack of reward/justice in terms of money, respect, job security leads to negative emotions ultimately leading to stress. The lack of motivation to perform comes from misplaced/improper resources. Both the factors contribute to eventual burn out, fatigue, depression and suicidal tendencies (Fig. **2**). Simulation studies have concluded that increasing job control and decreasing job demands led to decrease of workplace stress [4]. **ERI model reflect the current market sentiment stressful work environment and poor health of worker.** Workplace support and safety, work place-family conflict are other factors contributing stress. **Organizational Justice Model (OJ) was given in 1987 by Greenberg.** This model compliments JDC and ERI models as an index of social interaction. Fairness of decision making process, outcome and treatment by peers are three aspects of OJ model which have direct impact on workers

**Precarious Employment** has been on rise in recent decades owing to staggering economy worldwide, growing population and obsession of the heads of the states with defence expenditure. Standard employment opportunities comprising permanent, full time job with benefits is on decline. Though, precarious employment is much more common in relation to temporary employment particularly for women, young, migrant, minority worker. Underpaid and insecure employment which can not support a household is common amongst all classes of educated/uneducated, skilled/unskilled worker. A financially constrained worker is unlikely to have access to basic (housing, health,education), social and material comforts. Moreover, he/she is likely to work in hazardous work environment compromising health and safety standards culminating in job dissatisfaction-leading to poor mental health. Prolonged exposure to Precarious employment enhances chances of psychological stress further reducing a chance to secure a proper job. **Employment insecurity** forces a worker to continue job, in severe social and climatic conditions compromising on long working hours, lack of sanitation, untimely and low wages, without proper protective equipment (PPE), presenteeism (working while ill) resulting in anxiety and depression or a permanent injury/disease which plays havoc with **work-life balance.** Precarious employment, employment insecurity, often forces a person to take more than one job, sometimes work in two shifts affecting self health and adversely affecting family life. The disturbed work-life balance builds up further anxiety when employee is a parent too.

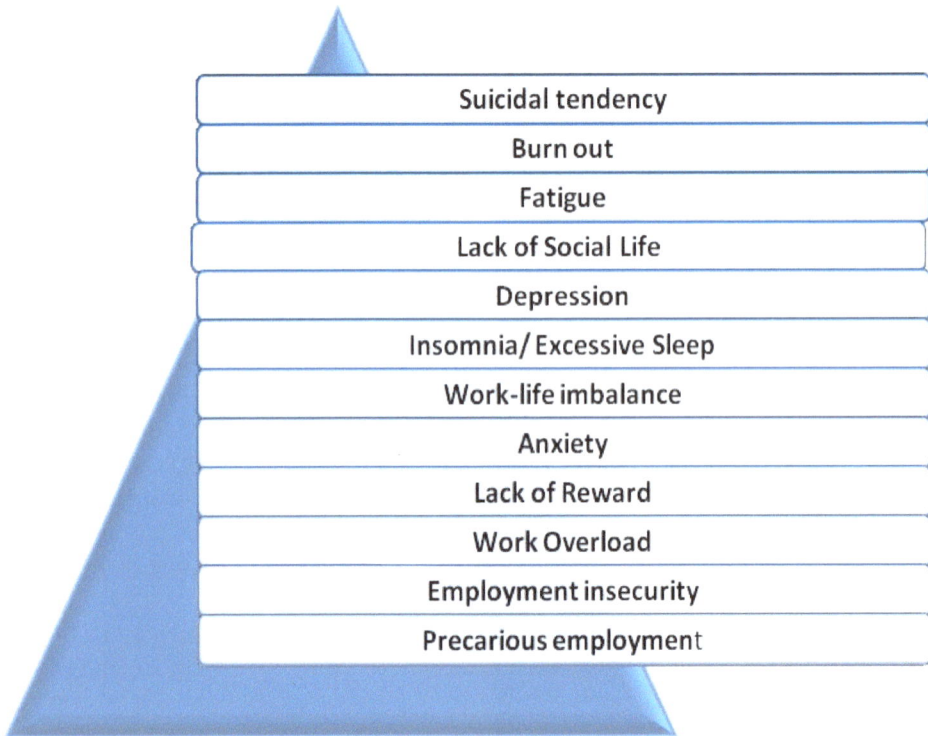

**Fig. (2).** Major contributors to stress.

## Key Role of Sleep Disruption in Building Stress

Sleep is important for the normal functioning of human body. The body repairs and regenerates itself during sleep. The quality and quantity of sleep which disrupt the continuity of sleep is called sleep disruption. The more the sleep disruptions, the lesser the work productivity as sleep loss disrupts attention and focus. Insomnia or lack of sleep is considered as a marker for mental health. An estimated 50-70 million Americans suffer from sleep related disorders and sleep wakefulness. The increased activity of SympatheticNervous system activates hypothalamic-pituitary-adrenal axis leading to Insomnia. *Sleep deprivation is not easily recognizable.* A study reports that patients of insomnia have higher levels of circulating Adrenocorticotropic Hormone (ACTH) and cortisol over a 24-hour period [5]. There are various effects of short term and long term sleep deprivation as summarized in Figs. (**3 & 4**). The workers who slept consistently poor had poor health and medical risk as compared to workers taking optimum sleep, thereby leading to poor productivity and high health costs [6]. Workplace violence also lead to sleep disruption if the perpetrator of violence is boss or a co-worker [7]. The organizations are encouraged by researchers to educate workers regarding sleep as a component of workers' health. There is a growing attitude towards taking around eight hours of daily sleep so as to allow the body to rest and repair.

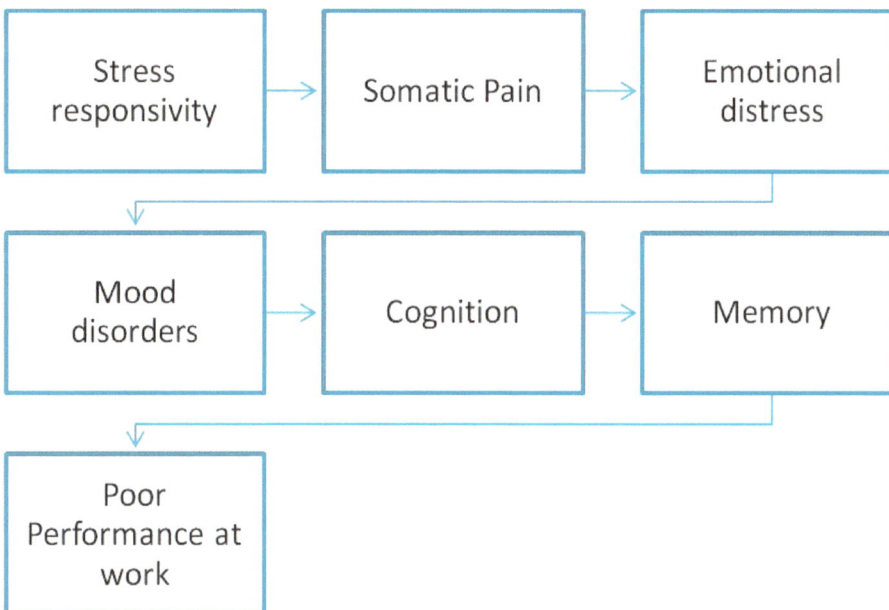

**Fig. (3).** Short term consequences of sleep deprivation.

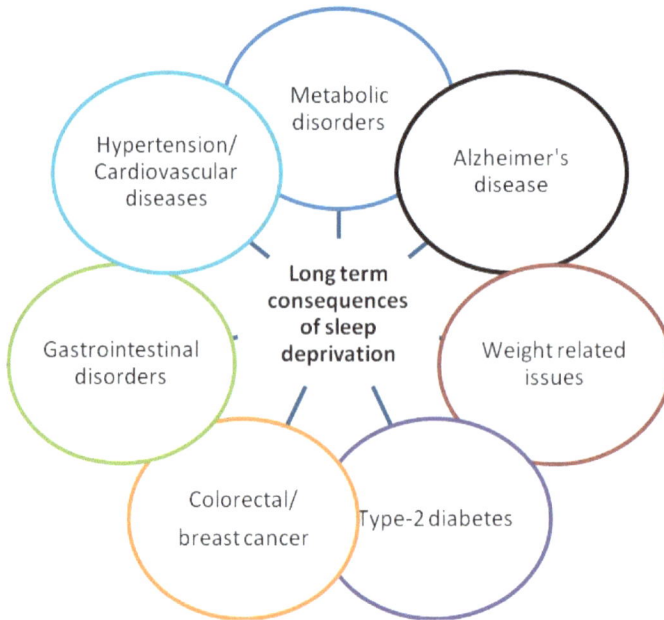

**Fig. (4).** Long term consequences of sleep deprivation.

## Molecular Mechanisms Behind Sleep

**Central body clock** is located in Suprachiasmatic Nucleus (SCN). It is a cluster of ≈ 2000 neurons in anterior hypothalamus while **peripheral clocks** are present in each and every tissue. The central and peripheral clocks work harmoniously to regulate Circadian rhythm. Circadian rhythms help organism to attain homeostasis with its environment through **clock genes.** There are clock genes in an organism which create a peak protein expression once every 24 hours to align it with solar day. **Period (per)** and **Timeless (tim)** are two clock genes regulated by negative feedback, whose products per and tim proteins ensure smooth metabolic process to create a precise Circadian rhythm. Suprachiasmatic Nucleus (SCN) receives brightness indications from nerve cells in retina; SCN signals pineal gland to secrete Melatonin.Clock Genes and Melatonin synchronize Circadian rhythm. Sleep-wake cycle is regulated through neurons in hypothalamus. Besides, sleep-wake cycle body temperature, blood pressure and hormonal secretion are also regulated through SCN-hypothalamus axis. The circadian rhythm collapses during ageing and disease; affecting endocrine and metabolic activities through autonomic nervous system and gut flora [8]. A cross sectional study concluded that high work stress leads to insomnia and the workers of *genotype AC*, an allele of clock gene called **per gene** are more susceptible to insomnia [9]. The *short term effect* of sleep deprivation leads to jet-lag-like- symptoms including fatigue, enhances blood pressure, impaired glycemic index and inflammation. On molecular level, sleep deprivation results in production of Reactive Oxygen species (ROS) which triggers metabolic problems and impairment of immune system [10].

*Long term chronic sleep deprivation* leads to decreased body weight, impaired learning and memory, declined motor function by triggering changes in prefrontal cortex pathways. The endocrine, neural and inflammatory long term effect of sleep deprivation result in Osteopenia (low bone mineral density) and Sarcopenia (low muscle mass) [11].

## Shift Work

Nursing, medical and paramedical staff, commercial vehicle drivers, airport and railway staff, hospitality industry workers, telecommunications, police and security agencies *work in shifts* to impart us a secure life. Latest studies conclude that shift work leads to insomnia or excessive sleepiness or both by disruption of circadian rhythm [12]. Circadian rhythm controls emotions, cognitive function and behaviour [8]; therefore, shift workers are more likely to face emotional, cognitive and behavioural issues. A study on Taiwanese workers revealed that fixed night shift is associated with greater sleep problems, greater chance of burnout and mental health issues [13]. Long work hours coupled with irregular shift lead to fatigue disturbing circadian rhythm [14], sleep quantity and quality which in turn lead to loss of focus and attention deficit culminating in accidents and injuries, deterioration in quality of work. Repeated disruption of sleep and night light leads to inhibition of pineal gland hormone, melatonin. Shift workers suffer from an array of abnormalities in sleep pattern like **delayed sleep phase disorder (DSPD)** due to suppression of secretion of *melatonin* owing to hypersensitivity of night time bright light [15]. Chronic insomnia, excessive sleepiness, impaired daytime functioning are characteristic of **delayed sleep phase disorder** in which there is stable delay of major sleep to the required sleep–wake time. Limited data from recent studies have suggested that shift workers have abnormal levels of circulating WBCsleading to immune system dysregulation [16]. Disruption of immune system is ultimately responsible for a wide number of disorders.

## Psychosocial Factors at Work

Workplace safety has become an important issue. Workplace bullying and politics is a common problem predominant in most professions including nursing staff. Collective gender bias pressurizes women at workstation irrespective of white collar or blue collar job. There are thousands of reported and unreported incidences about sexual abuse at work place. Violence against medical staff particularly physicians is common (Fig. **5**). In developing countries like India, both physical and verbal violence has been reported particularly at night, mostly with patients or their relatives [17]. Workplace support and safety, work place-family conflict are other psychosocial factors attributing stress. As the psychosocial hazards and work related stress have reached epidemic proportions in Europe, Italian law in 2008 made it obligatory for companies to assess work-related stress to ensure workers' safety and health [18].

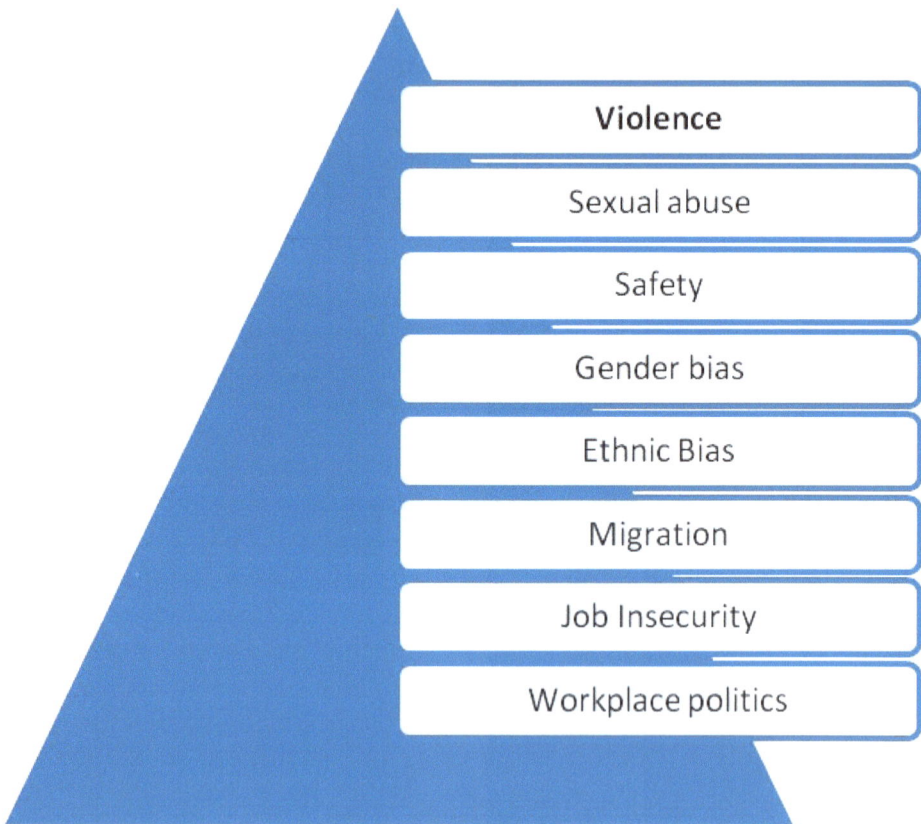

**Fig. (5).** Key Psychosocial factors at workplace contributing to stress.

## Migration

Global migrations are on rise. People migrate to newer geographic locations and countries in search of better work opportunities, with or without family (in case a person migrates with family, stress involves establishing at an altogether new location; other case of leaving the family, sometimes for years at stretch, is a stress in itself). Nursing profession is well-known for its demanding job and discriminatory behavior is vested out to migrant nurses particularly from India, Philippines, Europe and Africa. A systematic review revealed that migrant and minority nurses are at high risk of work-related injuries and discrimination than native or majority nurses [19]. The members of the *106th International Labour Conference* held on 5-16 June, 2017 inGeneva, Switzerland deliberated on work issues related to conflict and war zones and labour migration governance.

## Miscelleneous Work Stressors

The various work stressors are discussed in detail in Chapter 1. Thermal stress is an integrated part of work-place stress in some professions in both developed and developing economies. The heat stress could be indoor (like steel manufacturing) and outdoor (construction/agriculture) or cold stress indoor (like frozen food factories) and outdoor work (construction/ fishing/agriculture). *Noise and noise coupled with vibration* are well-recognized occupational hazards. Professional work like underwater archaeology, navy, and exploration for marine life, oil and natural gas may lead to Barotraumas due to compressed air. *Work related Musculoskeletal Disorders* (WRMSDs) cost a lot to the employer in terms of work quality and days/number of absent workers and employee in terms of reduced work days, cost of treatment and persistent pain. The quality of patients' life degrades and absentia from work enhances *after minor skin problems turn chronic*. Malodour at workplace due to environmental pollution leads to discomfort particularly in patients of post-traumatic stress [20]. Stress is a cause of major disorders.

Work related *anxiety* is related to development of hypertension in young adults [21]. *Anxiety and depression* have direct effects on work performance [22]. *Hypertension* (Fig. **6**) is an established work related risk particularly in white collar jobs [23]. In a comparative study on white and blue collar jobs, white collar jobs had significantly higher risk of *cardiovascular disease risk* [24]. Glycemic index is an indicator of early autonomic cardiac dysfunction indicated by a reduced heart rate variability [25]. The results of cross-sectional study on an industrial cohort indicated work-stress affects hypoglycemic index through heart rate variability as indicated by C-reactive protein leading to *Type-2 diabetes* [26]. A recent *case control* study showed that the Canadian workers with prolonged continued stress at workplace lead to *cancer* in 5 out of 11 cases [27]. The survivors of New York City (9/11) were exposed to intense dust of hazardous materials culminating in increased cases of *Asthma* and related respiratory diseases [28]. Job related injuries are common. An analysis revealed that workers with *permanent injury* are more prone to diseases and general health decline [29]. Some people resort to *alcoholism* due to its stimulant and sedative effects in response to work-related stress, but interventions are necessary to improve problematic heavy drinkers to ensure work place safety [30].

| | | | |
|---|---|---|---|
| Sleep disorders | Anxiety & Depression | Hyperstension &Cardiovascular Disease | Asthma |
| Cancer | Cognitive Impairment | Type-2 diabetes | Pain & Injury |
| | Alcoholism | Peridontitis | |

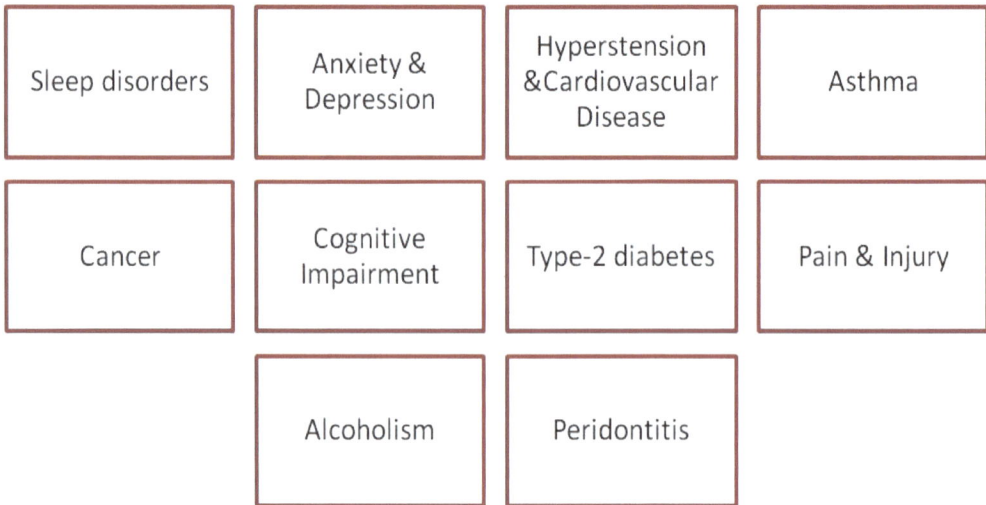

**Fig. (6).** Graphic list of some major stress related disorders.

## Mechanism of Chronic Emotional and Mental Stress

Stress negatively stimulates *hypothalamic-pituitary-adrenal axis and autonomic nervous system.* In order to maintain homeostasis, body requires adjustments or adaptations called allostasis. The term allostasis was coined by Sterling and Eyer in 1988 [31]. *Epinephrine, norepinephrine, cortisol, vagal tone etc. are called primary mediators* (Fig. **7**) *of allostasis* whose imbalance lead to Allostatic Load ensuing in **primary outcomes** like sleep disruption, anxiety, mood alteration. The cumulative effects of Allostatic overload result in **secondary outcomes** like inflammation, cold, cardiovascular risk *etc*. The dysregulation of **Allostatsis** ends in **tertiary outcomes** like cancer, depression, stroke, obesity, diabetes, Alzheimer's disease. **Allostatic Load Index (ALI)** developed by Seemans *et al*. in 1997 measures stress related wear and tear [32]. Chronic stress leads to hormonal disturbance disrupting the biological systems. ALI is a multicomponent measure of stress related health risk assessment among workers which indicates early impairment using physiological biomarkers. **Allostatic Load index (ALI)** encompasses as many as fifteen physiological parameters representing neuroendocrine, immune, metabolic and cardiovascular system dysfunctioning on chronological scale to predict stress induced loss of physical and mental health at work place. Waist to Hip Ratio (WHR), Body Mass Index (BMI), Systolic and diastolic blood pressure, Total Cholesterol, Triglycerides, **HDL (High Density Liporotein)** and **LDL (Low Density Liporotein)**, Total Thyroxine, Serum Cortisol, C-Reactive Protein, Dehydroepiandrosterone Sulphate (DHEA-S), Urinary epinephrine and norepinephrine are parameters taken into consideration for calculating **ALI**. A group of Canadian researchers hypothesised that higher ALI index represents higher stress, burnout symptoms as well as hypoactive diurnal and reactive stress hormone levels [33]. Diurnal variation in measure of cortisol level is an indicator of burnout and depression [34].

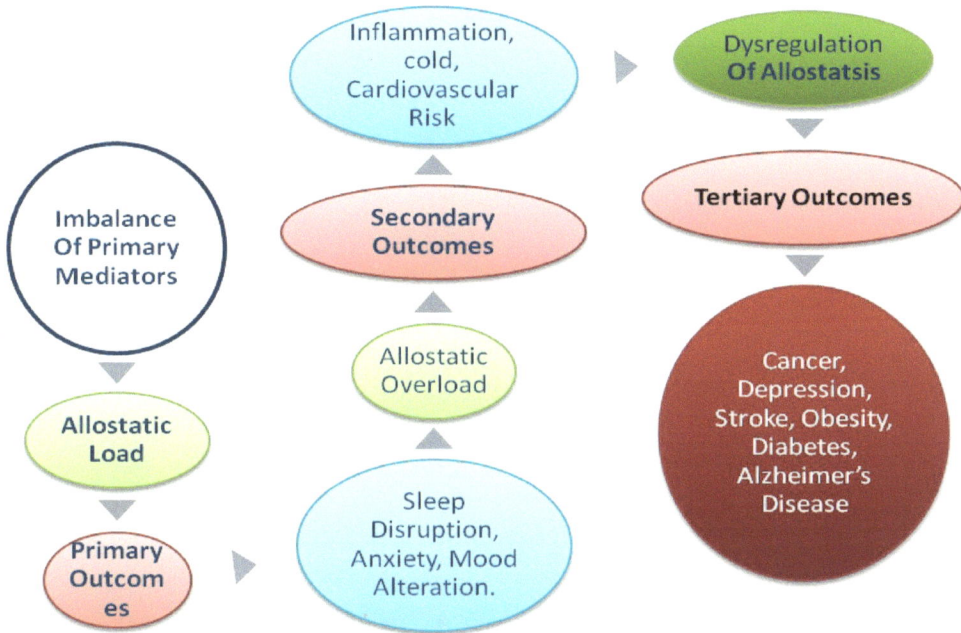

**Fig. (7).** Brief mechanism of chronic emotional and mental stress.

## Reducing Stress at Personal Level

Stress is a common problem. Though organizational support will definitely boast mental health, individual efforts to reduce stress will go a long way in improving quality of life. Social networking sites take a lot of precious time further depriving quality sleep and/or time that could have been well spent. Adequate sleep is a safe and healthy investment that repairs body preventing the onset of many diseases. The diagram below (Fig. **8**) suggests some measures to efficiently use leisure time so as to improve resilience and build up coping behavior.

## Role of Organisatons in Maintaining Mental Health

Work-related suicides and depression are a reality. Even the person with the weakest disposition does not commit suicide instantaneously. It takes long hours of contemplation to finally take the drastic step. Some occupations, some societies are emotionally too weak to prevent the final undesirable step; for instance, in male dominated construction industry, suicide is very high in Australian construction workers due to a number of work (inability to get proper job, work-place injury, chronic illness) and non work factors (substance abuse, marital disputes, *etc.*) [35]. Coping behavior in relation to suicidal tendencies are gender sensitive as demonstrated by studies on Japanese people with a high rate of suicide [36]. Reduction of work stressors led to decrease in suicidal thoughts in Chinese petroleum industry workers [37].

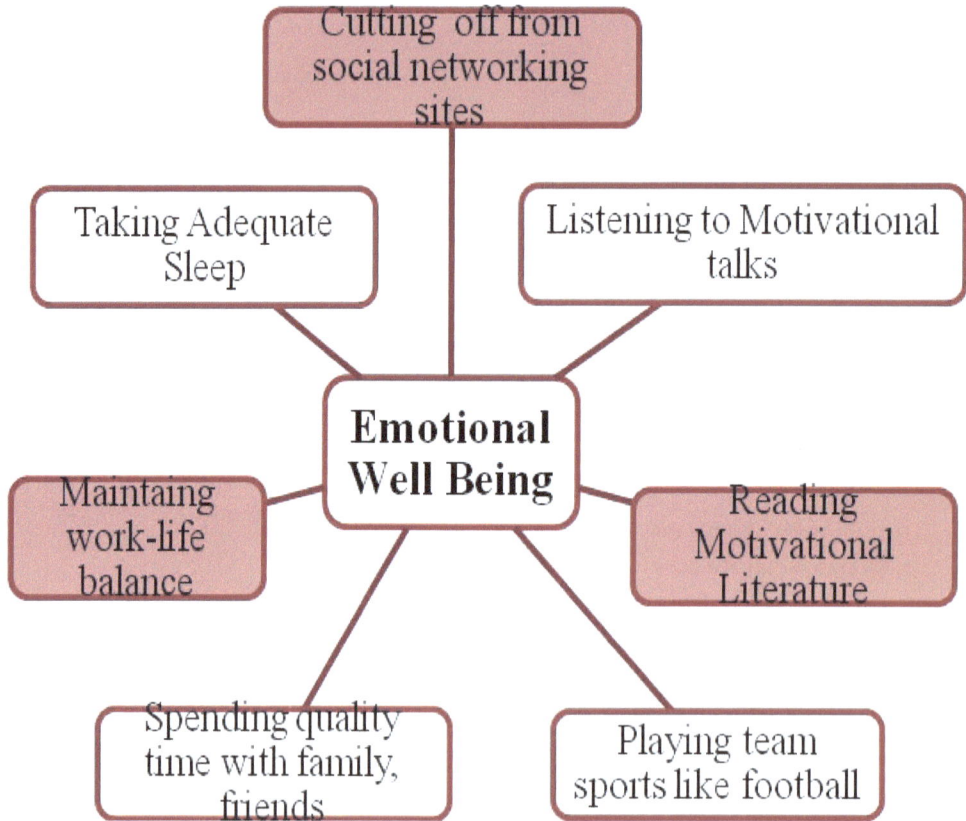

**Fig. (8).** Ideas for maintaining emotional wellbeing.

## CONCLUSION

Change in work stressors is now viewed as a preventive measure to reduce suicidal tendencies (Fig. **9**). Organizations are being advised to consider providing health support to their workers as productivity and welfare of workers are inter-related [38]. All the associations worldwide try to retain valued employees by giving them paid maternity leave or bonuses. Similarly, all the Organizations should try to reduce stress induced burn out in workers. Over-stressed professional might consider leaving the job or harming self. The organizations should take care of their pool of talent and skill by taking the following measures. They might consider avoiding work at odd hours, reducing work load and ensure workplace safety (from violence, sexual abuse, gender bias and office politics). The organization of motivational talks, mindfulness based wellness programs and counseling sessions might reduce work related stress. Reward, fair chance, values coupled by resilience on part of the employer also reduced stress in child protection workers of Ireland [39]. It is reported that introduction of Meditation, Yoga,Tai Chi and Quiong had positive impact on workers in US [40]. Patients on sick leave suffering from prolonged work related stress were found to be sleep deprived and cognitively impaired in a longitudinal study, the study also concluded that reduction in work related stress reversed initial cognitive decline and insomnia [41]. The rise in number of chronic diseases among shift workers can be decreased if the workers take healthy diet and improve their dietary practices [42]. **Besides these measures, adequate sleep is just like basic practice of sanitation and hygiene which if properly practiced averts a lot of maladies.**

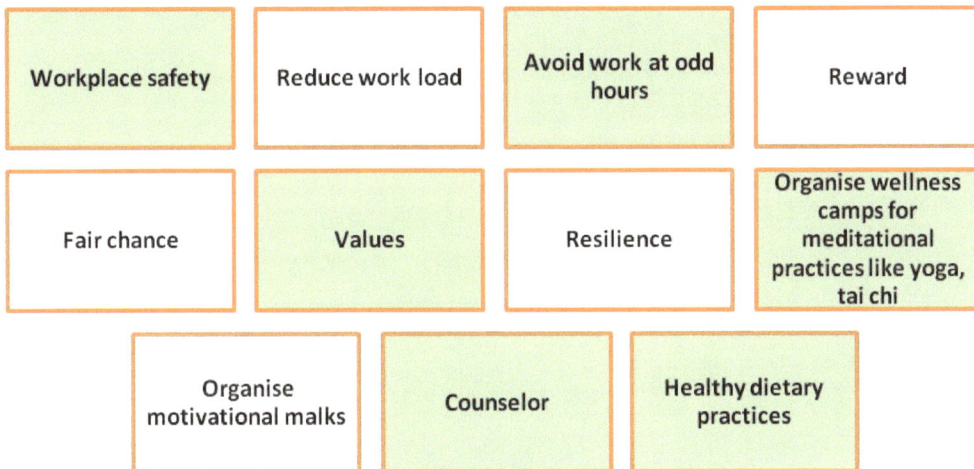

**Fig. (9).** Alteration of work stressors that can bring positive outcome.

## CONSENT FOR PUBLICATION

Not applicable.

## ACKNOWLEDGEMENTS

Declared none

## CONFLICT OF INTEREST

The author confirms that this chapter contents have no conflict of interest.

# REFERENCES

[1]     González ER, Irastorza WCX. ESENER - European survey of enterprises on new and emerging risks. European risk observatory report. Managing safety and health at work 2010. http://osha.europa.eu

[2]     Vander Elst T, Cavents C, Daneels K, *et al.* Job demands-resources predicting burnout and work engagement among Belgian home health care nurses: A cross-sectional study. Nurs Outlook 2016; 64(6): 542-56.
[http://dx.doi.org/10.1016/j.outlook.2016.06.004] [PMID: 27427405]

[3]     Losa Iglesias ME, Becerro de Bengoa Vallejo R, Salvadores Fuentes P. The relationship between experiential avoidance and burnout syndrome in critical care nurses: a cross-sectional questionnaire survey. Int J Nurs Stud 2010; 47(1): 30-7.
[http://dx.doi.org/10.1016/j.ijnurstu.2009.06.014] [PMID: 19625023]

[4]     Jetha A, Kernan L, Kurowski A. Conceptualizing the dynamics of workplace stress: a systems-based study of nursing aides. BMC Health Serv Res 2017; 17(1): 12.
[http://dx.doi.org/10.1186/s12913-016-1955-8] [PMID: 28056973]

[5]     Vgontzas AN, Bixler EO, Lin HM, *et al.* Chronic insomnia is associated with nyctohemeral activation of the hypothalamic-pituitary-adrenal axis: clinical implications. J Clin Endocrinol Metab 2001; 86(8): 3787-94.
[http://dx.doi.org/10.1210/jcem.86.8.7778] [PMID: 11502812]

[6]     Chen CY, Schultz AB, Li X, Burton WN. The association between changes in employee sleep and changes in workplace health and economic outcomes. Popul Health Manag 2017. Epub ahead of print
[http://dx.doi.org/10.1089/pop.2016.0169] [PMID: 28486056]

[7]     Yoo T, Ye B, Kim JI, Park S. Relationship of workplace violence and perpetrators on sleep disturbance - data from the 4th Korean working conditions survey. Ann Occup Environ Med 2016; 19(28): 59.

[8]     Futamura A, Shiromaru A, Kuroda T, *et al.* Brainclocks, behavior, and cognition. Brain Nerve 2017; 69(6): 639-49.
[http://dx.doi.org/10.11477/mf.1416200795] [PMID: 28596466]

[9]     Li J, Huang C, Lan Y, Wang Y. A cross-sectional study on the relationships among the polymorphism of period2 gene, work stress, and insomnia. Sleep Breath 2015; 19(4): 1399-406.
[http://dx.doi.org/10.1007/s11325-015-1229-4] [PMID: 26174845]

[10]    Haus EL, Smolensky MH. Shift work and cancer risk: potential mechanistic roles of circadian disruption, light at night, and sleep deprivation. Sleep Med Rev 2013; 17(4): 273-84.
[http://dx.doi.org/10.1016/j.smrv.2012.08.003] [PMID: 23137527]

[11]    Lucassen EA, de Mutsert R, le Cessie S, *et al.* Poor sleep quality and later sleep timing are risk factors for osteopenia and sarcopenia in middle-aged men and women: The NEO study. PLoS One 2017; 12(5): e0176685.
[http://dx.doi.org/10.1371/journal.pone.0176685] [PMID: 28459884]

[12]    Wickwire EM. Geiger-Brown J, Scharf SM, Drake CL. Shift work and shift works leep disorder: clinical and organizational perspectives. Chest 2017; 151(5): 1156-72.
[http://dx.doi.org/10.1016/j.chest.2016.12.007] [PMID: 28012806]

[13]    Cheng WJ, Cheng Y. Night shift and rotating shift in association with sleep problems, burnout and minor mental disorder in male and female employees. Occup Environ Med 2017; 74(7): 483-8.
[http://dx.doi.org/10.1136/oemed-2016-103898] [PMID: 27810939]

[14]    Santhi N, Duffy JF, Horowitz TS, Czeisler CA. Scheduling of sleep/darkness affects the circadian phase of night shift workers. Neurosci Lett 2005; 384(3): 316-20.
[http://dx.doi.org/10.1016/j.neulet.2005.04.094] [PMID: 15919151]

[15]    Czeisler CA, Richardson GS, Zimmerman JC, Moore-Ede MC, Weitzman ED. Entrainment of human circadian rhythms by light-dark cycles: a reassessment. Photochem Photobiol 1981; 34(2): 239-47.

[http://dx.doi.org/10.1111/j.1751-1097.1981.tb09354.x] [PMID: 7267730]

[16]     Wirth MD, Andrew ME, Burchfiel CM, *et al.* Association of shiftwork and immune cells among police officers from the Buffalo Cardio-Metabolic Occupational Police Stress study. Chronobiol Int 2017; 34(6): 721-31.
[http://dx.doi.org/10.1080/07420528.2017.1316732] [PMID: 28488901]

[17]     Kumar M, Verma M, Das T, Pardeshi G, Kishore J, Padmanandan A. A study of workplace violence experienced by doctors and associated risk factors in a tertiary care hospital of South Delhi, India. J Clin Diagn Res 2016; 10(11): LC06-10.
[PMID: 28050406]

[18]     De Sio S, Cedrone F, Greco E, *et al.* Job stress: an in-depth investigation based on the HSE questionnaire and a multistep approach in order to identify the most appropriate corrective actions. Clin Ter 2016; 167(6): e143-9.
[http://dx.doi.org/10.7417/CT.2016.1959] [PMID: 28051827]

[19]     Schilgen B, Nienhaus A, Handtke O, Schulz H, Mösko M. Health situation of migrant and minority nurses: A systematic review. PLoS One 2017; 12(6): e0179183.
[http://dx.doi.org/10.1371/journal.pone.0179183]

[20]     Tjalvin G, Magerøy N, Bråtveit M, Lygre SH, Hollund BE, Moen BE. Odour as a determinant of persistent symptoms after a chemical explosion, a longitudinal study. Ind Health 2017 Jul; 55(2): 127.: 137.

[21]     Mucci N, Giorgi G, De Pasquale Ceratti S, Fiz-Pérez J, Mucci F, Arcangeli G. Anxiety, stress-related factors, and blood pressure in young adults. Front Psychol 2016; 7: 1682. eCollection 2016

[22]     Ivandic I, Kamenov K, Rojas D, Cerón G, Nowak D, Sabariego C. Determinants of work performance in workers with depression and anxiety: A cross-sectional study. Int J Environ Res Public Health 2017; 14(5): E466.
[http://dx.doi.org/10.3390/ijerph14050466] [PMID: 28445433]

[23]     Boucher P, Gilbert-Ouimet M, Trudel X, Duchaine CS, Milot A, Brisson C. Masked hypertension and effort-reward imbalance at work among 2369 white-collar workers. J Hum Hypertens 2017; 31(10): 620-6.
[http://dx.doi.org/10.1038/jhh.2017.42] [PMID: 28639611]

[24]     Aginsky KD, Constantinou D, Delport M, Watson ED. Cardiovascular disease risk profile and readiness to change in blue- and white-collar workers. Fam Community Health 2017; 40(3): 236-44.
[http://dx.doi.org/10.1097/FCH.0000000000000148] [PMID: 28525444]

[25]     Jaiswal M, Fingerlin TE, Urbina EM, *et al.* Impact of glycemic control on heart rate variability in youth with type 1 diabetes: the SEARCH CVD study. Diabetes Technol Ther 2013; 15(12): 977-83.
[http://dx.doi.org/10.1089/dia.2013.0147] [PMID: 24010960]

[26]     Jarczok MN, Koenig J, Li J, *et al.* The association of work stress and glycemic status is partially mediated by autonomic nervous system function: cross-sectional results from the Mannheim Industrial Cohort Study (MICS). PLoS One 2016; 11(8): e0160743.
[http://dx.doi.org/10.1371/journal.pone.0160743] [PMID: 27532642]

[27]     Blanc-Lapierre A, Rousseau MC, Weiss D, El-Zein M, Siemiatycki J, Parent MÉ. Lifetime report of perceived stress at work and cancer among men: A case-control study in Montreal, Canada. Prev Med 2017; 96: 28-35.
[http://dx.doi.org/10.1016/j.ypmed.2016.12.004] [PMID: 27923666]

[28]     Alper HE, Yu S, Stellman SD, Brackbill RM. Injury, intense dust exposure, and chronic disease among survivors of the World Trade Center terrorist attacks of September 11, 2001. Inj Epidemiol 2017; 4(1): 17.
[http://dx.doi.org/10.1186/s40621-017-0115-x] [PMID: 28626847]

[29]     Casey R, Ballantyne PJ. Diagnosed chronic health conditions among injured workers with permanent

impairments and the general population. Psychol Health 2017; 32(8): 976-1017.
[http://dx.doi.org/10.1080/08870446.2017.1325889] [PMID: 28513195]

[30]    Frone MR. Work stress and alcohol use: Developing and testing a biphasic self-medication model. Work Stress 2016; 30(4): 374-94.
[http://dx.doi.org/10.1080/02678373.2016.1252971] [PMID: 28090129]

[31]    Sterling P, Eyer J. Handbook of life stress, cognition and health Allostasis: a new paradigm to explain arousal pathology. New York: John Wiley & Sons 1988; pp. 629-49.

[32]    Seeman TE, Singer BH, Rowe JW, Horwitz RI, McEwen BS. Price of adaptation--allostatic load and its health consequences. MacArthur studies of successful aging. Arch Intern Med 1997; 157(19): 2259-68.
[http://dx.doi.org/10.1001/archinte.1997.00440400111013] [PMID: 9343003]

[33]    Juster RP, Sindi S, Marin MF, *et al.* A clinical allostatic load index is associated with burnout symptoms and hypocortisolemic profiles in healthy workers. Psychoneuroendocrinology 2011; 36(6): 797-805.
[http://dx.doi.org/10.1016/j.psyneuen.2010.11.001] [PMID: 21129851]

[34]    Marchand A, Durand P, Juster RP, Lupien SJ. Workers' psychological distress, depression, and burnout symptoms: associations with diurnal cortisol profiles. Scand J Work Environ Health 2014; 40(3): 305-14.
[http://dx.doi.org/10.5271/sjweh.3417] [PMID: 24469265]

[35]    Milner A, Maheen H, Currier D, LaMontagne AD. Male suicide among construction workers in Australia: a qualitative analysis of the major stressors precipitating death. BMC Public Health 2017; 17(1): 584.
[http://dx.doi.org/10.1186/s12889-017-4500-8] [PMID: 28629352]

[36]    Sugawara N, Yasui-Furukori N, Sasaki G, *et al.* Coping behaviors in relation to depressive symptoms and suicidal ideation among middle-aged workers in Japan. J Affect Disord 2012; 142(1-3): 264-8.
[http://dx.doi.org/10.1016/j.jad.2012.05.011] [PMID: 22835844]

[37]    Xiao J, Guan S, Ge H, *et al.* The impact of changes in work stressors and coping resources on the risk of new-onset suicide ideation among Chinese petroleum industry workers. J Psychiatr Res 2017; 88: 1-8. Epub ahead of print
[http://dx.doi.org/10.1016/j.jpsychires.2016.12.014] [PMID: 28043011]

[38]    Rothermund E, Kilian R, Rottler E, *et al.* Improving access to mental health care by delivering psychotherapeutic care in the workplace: A cross-sectional exploratory trial. PLoS One 2017; 12(1): e0169559.
[http://dx.doi.org/10.1371/journal.pone.0169559] [PMID: 28056101]

[39]    McFadden P, Mallett J, Leiter M. Extending the two-process model of burnout in child protection workers: The role of resilience in mediating burnout via organizational factors of control, values, fairness, reward, workload, and community relationships. Stress Health 2018; 34(1): 72-83.
[http://dx.doi.org/10.1002/smi.2763] [PMID: 28544380]

[40]    Kachan D, Olano H, Tannenbaum SL, *et al.* Prevalence of mindfulness practices in the US workforce: national health interview survey. Prev Chronic Dis 2017; 14: E01.
[http://dx.doi.org/10.5888/pcd14.160034] [PMID: 28055821]

[41]    Eskildsen A, Fentz HN, Andersen LP, Pedersen AD, Kristensen SB, Andersen JH. Perceived stress, disturbed sleep, and cognitive impairments in patients with work-related stress complaints: a longitudinal study. Stress 2017; 20(4): 371-8.
[http://dx.doi.org/10.1080/10253890.2017.1341484] [PMID: 28605986]

[42]    Ferri GM, Cavone D, Intranuovo G, Macinagrossa L. Healthy diet and reduction of chronic disease risks of night shiftworkers. Curr Med Chem 2017.
[http://dx.doi.org/10.2174/0929867324666170720160632] [PMID: 28730970]

# SUBJECT INDEX

## A

Abortion, spontaneous 93, 94, 101, 106
Absorption 68, 71
Acquired 7, 87, 90, 91, 115, 132, 134, 153, 154, 136
  immunodeficiency syndrome (AIDS) 87, 90, 91, 136
  infections 7, 115, 132, 134, 153, 154
Acremonium sp 8, 9
Acute respiratory infections (ARI) 87, 95
Adenovirus vectors 139
Adrenocorticotropic hormone (ACTH) 162
Advisory committee on immunization practices (ACIP) 135
Aerodynamic diameter 67
Aerosol generation 131, 132, 133, 136
  procedures 133
Aerosols 7, 9, 90, 92, 119, 126, 130, 132, 135, 136
Aflatoxin 8, 69
Agents 1, 4, 6, 7, 29, 30, 31, 44, 62, 63, 64, 65, 70, 76, 78, 83, 85, 90, 99, 103, 106, 122, 125, 129, 130, 131, 138, 139, 147, 149, 150
  alkylating 70, 76
  cancer-causing 62, 63
  carcinogenic 83
  causing occupational cancer 76
  chemical/physical 76
  infectious 1, 7, 90, 129, 130, 149, 150
  non-infectious 150
Airway sensitisation 2, 25
Alkalis 118, 124, 143, 148
Allergens 29, 31, 149
Allergic 28, 29, 30, 31, 106
  contact dermatitis (ACD) 28, 29, 30, 31
  reaction 106
Allostatic load 167
Allostatsis 158, 167
Alzheimer's disease 41, 43, 45, 48, 49, 50, 158, 167
Amoebiasis 99
Anaesthetic drugs 87
Aniline 64, 78, 80
  dye workers 64
Animals 9, 24, 99, 100, 122, 131, 139, 140, 149, 150, 153

bedding 149, 150
carcasses 149
infected 99, 100, 140
Anti-neoplastic drugs 105, 106
Antisepsis 108, 110
Anxiety, accumulating 158, 160
Arsenic 11, 31, 44, 47, 48, 49, 64, 151
  exposure to 48, 49
  high levels of 48
  median concentration of 48
Asbestos 26, 64, 66, 70, 75, 78, 84
*Aspergillus sp* 8, 9
Asthma 24, 28, 106, 118, 166
  occupational 24, 106
Autoclave 114, 122, 125, 126, 149, 151, 154
Autopsy 133

## B

Benzene 3, 31, 64, 68, 76, 78, 80
Biohazard 87, 102, 103, 130, 137
  levels 87, 102, 103
Biological agents 1, 4, 6, 7, 69, 114, 122, 138, 151, 152
  of disease 7
Biological
  expression systems 138
  hazards 19, 90, 115, 116
  materials 88, 114, 150, 153
  properties 138
  safety cabinet (BSC) 116, 123, 125, 126, 127, 128
  safety levels (BSL) 102, 122, 130, 138, 139, 140, 141, 147
Biological wastes 149, 150, 151, 152, 153
  infectious 150
Biosafety 102, 114, 115, 122, 126, 130, 131, 136, 137, 138, 139, 142, 153, 154
  cabinets 122, 126, 130, 136, 154
Biosecurity 114, 127, 137, 153
Bioterrorism agent 133

Bites, mosquito 88, 100, 102
Blood 13, 16, 17, 67, 68, 97, 116, 118, 131, 132, 142, 143, 144, 149, 152, 163
  animal 131, 142, 149, 152
  -borne pathogens (BBP) 116, 131

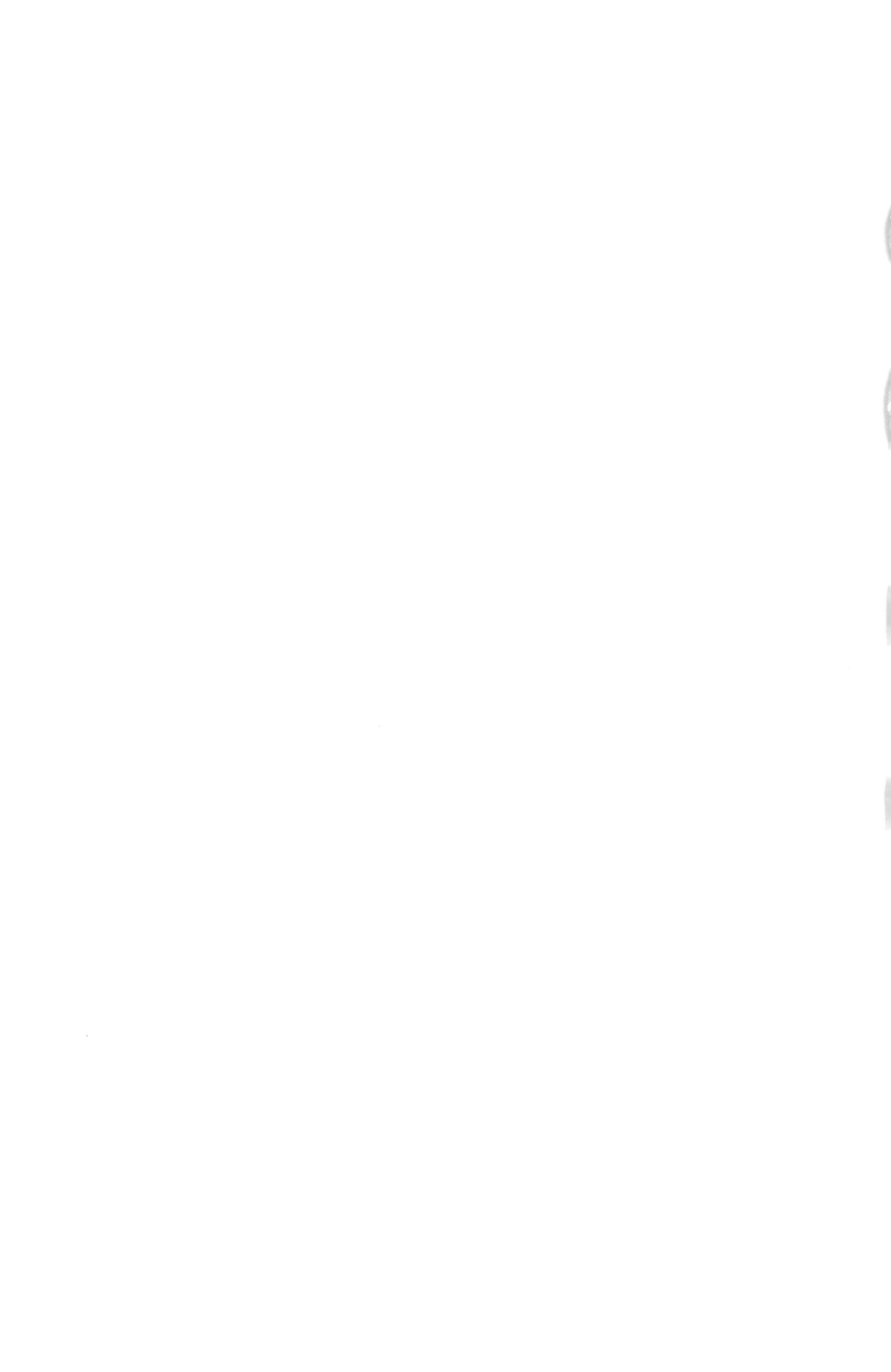

www.ingramcontent.com/pod-product-compliance
Lightning Source LLC
Chambersburg PA
CBHW041701210326
41598CB00007B/495